SEX, LIES & STDs
THE MUST READ BEFORE YOU SWIPE RIGHT

Rob Huizenga, MD
with Jeffrey Klausner, MD, MPH

Einsteinium - 99

ACKNOWLEDGMENTS

Much appreciation for each and every talented contributor.

Adoni Vrykoakas - Medical illustrator

Doctors Cornelis Rietmeijer, Uttam Sinha, Jeffrey Klausner and Rob Huizenga - Medical pictures

Sue Douglas and Jennifer Cole - Graphic design and layout of book and covers

Linda Huizenga and Claudia Sloan - Medical editors

Claudia Sloan and Candis Melamed - Thanks for the late save

Raquel - Thanks for tolerating all the weird looks our friends gave when they saw stacks of STD articles littered in every corner of the house

Table of Contents

Table of Contents – STD Capsule Summaries

FOREWORD

I first met Dr. Robert J. Huizenga in the wee hours of a now-infamous January night in 2011. He was the attending physician on call in the initial phase of what I like to refer to as *"The hernia heard 'round the world,"* but that's a different story, for some other moment in time.

He was holding a chart, a stethoscope and a mean-looking Foley catheter. In hindsight, I wish instead he'd been holding a copy of this very book.

Dr. H, as he's known to friends and colleagues alike, has been in the earliest HIV trenches and on the frontlines from ground-zero to patient-zero to today's most promising breakthroughs.

His tireless steadfast research in concert with his unrivaled compassion and intellect brings to birth a *"Manual of Arm's"* to these insidious life-and-death realities we ALL must bear witness to.

Never before has a more detailed and medically corroborated collection of the truth existed in a singular publication. I encourage one and all to invest the time absorbing what awaits you on the following pages.

Perhaps unlike myself, you can avoid that dreaded moment down the line, when a doctor says to you, "Your results are in. You might want to take a seat."

Respectfully and with gratitude,

Charlie Sheen

CHAPTER 1
Sexually Transmitted Diseases (STDs):
Tiny Pathogens, Big Problems

It was the best of times, it was the worst of times, it was the age of wisdom, it was the age of foolishness... Like this classic Charles Dickens opening sentence, the global STD epidemic readily lends itself to opposing hyperbole.

Unprecedented scientific advances have finally given us the tools to wipe STDs off the face of the earth! We can now readily diagnose and cure gonorrhea, chlamydia, syphilis, hepatitis C and pubic lice — merciless STDs that have plagued men and women since the beginning of time. We can now see incredible results from brand new human immunodeficiency virus, human papillomavirus and Hepatitis B prevention approaches. We can now finally accurately diagnose and treat mycoplasma and herpes.

Shockingly, these innovative anti-STD measures are for the most part falling on deaf ears! HIV and herpes are slightly decreasing, but other STDs show alarmingly steep increases. On August 28, 2018, the CDC reported gonorrhea, syphilis and chlamydia had increased by a whopping 67, 76 and 21 percent respectively in just the last four years to all time highs! And in urban areas, debilitating neonatal syphilis had increased 600 percent.

The overall picture is similarly dreadful. Over 145 million Americans are currently living with an active STD.

An equally appalling 3.3 billion individuals worldwide are currently living with one of these STDs.

The STD epidemic is fanned by one critical fact: the majority of infected individuals are completely unaware! They're oblivious! They have no clue that at this very moment, they are contagious!

TOP 10 STDS, CURRENT INFECTIONS (U.S.)

		Current Cases, U.S.
Human Papilloma Virus (HPV)		79,000,000
Genital Herpes Simplex Virus (adult onset)		55,000,000
HSV1 – oral (adult onset)	35,000,000	
HSV1 - genital	25,000,000	
HSV2 - genital	30,000,000	
Chlamydia		1,800,000
Mycoplasma		1,700,000
Trichomonas		3,700,000
Gonorrhea		250,000
Pubic Lice		120,000
Syphilis		120,000
Hepatitis		3,920,000
Hep C	3,500,000	
Hep B	420,000	
Human Immunodeficiency Virus (HIV)		1,100,000
TOTAL CURRENT STD CASES (U.S.)		**145 Million**

Table 1

TOP 10 STDS, CURRENT INFECTIONS (WORLD)

		Current Cases, World
Human Papilloma Virus (HPV)		1,800,000,000
Herpes Simplex Virus (adult onset)		780,000,000
HSV1 – oral (adult)	140,000,000	
HSV1 - genital	140,000,000	
HSV2 - genital	500,000,000	
Chlamydia		130,000,000
Mycoplasma		Unknown
Trichomonas		100,000,000
Gonorrhea		27,000,000
Pubic Lice		Unknown
Syphilis		18,000,000
Hepatitis		400,000,000
Hep C	140,000,000	
Hep B	260,000,000	
Human Immunodeficiency Virus (HIV)		37,000,000
TOTAL CURRENT STD CASES (WORLD)		**3.3 Billion**

Table 2

They register for online dating apps like Tinder, Match.com or Grindr. (Probably the most aptly named dating app ever!) They go to their local saloon, fly to Vegas, vacation in L.A. or go stand in line to get into *Catch*, Hollywood's current hottest celebrity watering hole. (Definitely the most aptly named nightclub ever!)

But what happens when you mix one part of each of the following trends: dating apps, nightclubs, lack of sex-ed, decreasing condom usage, STD confusion, and an impotent, politicized public health system?

You get the perfect storm to catch an STD. This year alone, 25 million Americans will catch an STD!

Catch an STD
#10 This year, 31,000 Americans will catch hepatitis C; 19,000 will catch Hepatitis B.
#9 This year, 38,000 Americans will catch human immunodeficiency virus (HIV).
#8 This year, 88,000 Americans will catch syphilis.
#7 This year, 120,000 Americans will catch pubic lice (crabs).
#6 This year, 820,000 Americans will catch gonorrhea.
#5 This year, 1,100,000 Americans will catch trichomoniasis.
#4 This year, 2,800,000 Americans will catch mycoplasma.
#3 This year, 2,900,000 Americans will catch chlamydia.
#2 This year, 3,000,000 American adults will catch herpes - herpes simplex 1 (1,600,000) or herpes simplex 2 (1,400,000).
#1 This year, 14,000,000 Americans will catch genital human papilloma virus (HPV).

Table 3

The new game changer? Anonymous sex.

Online dating has fueled nameless hook-ups. Popular sites facilitate billions of matches among persons that in the recent past, would have had little, if any chance of meeting. Resultant casual sex is occurring more frequently among partners who might only exchange online "handles," keeping full names and residences confidential. That is the death knell for old school STD control! Remember when public health officials could notify partners? Even STD positives, willing to cooperate, often have no identifying information of their recent partners!

Without notification, infected partners typically go untreated. Few persons have any idea exactly what early STD symptoms to look out for, even if symptoms did occur, because... spoiler alert... the most likely way an STD occurs is with *no symptoms whatsoever!*

Talk about silent but deadly!

Spoiler alert...

The most likely presentation of an STD is no symptoms whatsoever! Talk about silent but deadly!

Despite an "unlimited" amount of searchable internet topics, accurate user-friendly STD information is near impossible to find. What's the exact chance of contracting each STD? Does the chance of transmission differ between vaginal or anal sex? Can you get STDs with oral sex? What STDs can you get non-sexually? How long after STD transmission are tests able to detect the infection? Can condoms stop all STDs? If not, what's the best prevention?

I'm a Harvard trained doctor - and I couldn't easily find these answers!

We're awash in STD misconceptions. Come on. It's time to set the record straight.

First, we must de-stigmatize sexually transmitted diseases. Be honest. STDs are a normal part of being sexually active, just as a bruise, sprain or strain is a normal consequence of being physically active. In the majority of instances, STDs are not a sign of promiscuous or "morally bad" behavior. *There is no shame in contracting an STD.* The tragedy is when a lack of awareness leads to needless spread and complications from easily treatable infections!

Last weekend at a dinner party, someone asked me what I was up to – I said "writing a book about STDs." Big mistake. Everyone's ears picked up but believe me, nothing takes the air out of a dinner party faster than voicing an opinion about genital herpes or bacterial vaginosis. STDs are tabooer table conversation than either politics or religion!

Finally, one woman said what all were thinking, "STDs are *so* scary!"

"No," I replied, "When you protect yourself, STDs are no big deal. What's scary is ignorance and inaction!"

STDs are so scary!

*No they're not! When you protect yourself,
STDs are no big deal. What's scary is ignorance
and inaction!*

Second, let's identify the millions of Americans who have no idea they're infected. Let's designate September *STD awareness month* and all get screened together, stopping the vicious cycle of symptom-less persons continuing to spread STDs. Surprisingly, even individuals at high risk (men who have sex with men, heterosexuals with multiple partners, sex workers, IV drug users) tend to do routine STD checks far less than the minimal once a year recommendation.

Third, let's teach comprehensive STD prevention. Condoms, when used properly, work well but they are not a panacea. They provide at best 80 percent protection for HIV, syphilis and chlamydia, but only 50 percent protection for viruses spread thru genital skin like HPV and herpes and no protection for STDs like pubic lice and genital herpes type 1. Additional measures are necessary. Vaccination — before STD exposure — is of course the goal.

So yes, we must invest in our sexual health by fast tracking syphilis, gonorrhea, chlamydia, herpes and HIV vaccine development — the fourth cornerstone to counter the STD "catch" epidemic. But for now, we must fully utilize *the new prevention. Treatment.* Prioritizing the identification and full treatment of all those who are silently infected is today's best solution to this 145-million-person morass!

Sounds simple, huh? Only until you've run headlong into the barricades protecting the status quo in the U.S. As you can imagine, STD education is an uphill battle when the president of the United States twice asks Bill Gates if there is any difference between HIV and HPV. Some university medical "experts" seem just as confused. They recommend persons at risk not test for diseases like herpes, which is most often silent, because of the potential "emotional" harm of incorrect diagnoses by out-of-touch doctors who order old, inaccurate diagnostic tests.

Other misconceptions exist as well. Nearly a fourth of American adults are suspicious of vaccines – an intervention with a stellar balance of benefits to risks. Millions believe STDs present with obvious tell-tale symptoms. Millions naively shave pubic hair the same day they anticipate having sexual contact.

Millions lie to their partners. Half of all men and two-thirds of women believe they have been lied to for purposes of sex. Half of both men and women lie and understate the number of previous sex partners. Four-fifths of men and two-thirds of women would not initially disclose a single episode of sexual infidelity. Inaccurate and stigmatizing expose's about "celebrity's" STDs are frequently reported.

Ouch. Are we still in the Dark Ages when it comes to sex and STDs? Sex is a natural, fun and healthy part of our life. How did half-truths, ignorance and outright lies about common but preventable STDs become so damn widespread? I've seen lots of inaccurate media reports about celebrity patients over the years, but nothing prepared me for the ignorance I witnessed after Charlie Sheen's *Today Show* revelation.

Perhaps then, an appropriate place to start is when he and Matt Lauer went toe-to-toe...

CHAPTER 2
Matt Lauer Toe-to-Toe With
Hollywood Bad Boy, Charlie Sheen
Dateline: November 17, 2015. 8 a.m. EST. Rockefeller Center,
New York City

It was one of the most eagerly anticipated interviews in the more than 50-year history of NBC's *Today Show*. Host Matt Lauer toe-to-toe with comedy genius slash Hollywood bad boy Charlie Sheen on America's most popular daytime talk show. Lauer was set to confirm an explosive story that had been building like a Mt. St. Helen's-sized volcano in the tabloids for months — and I had a front row seat.

The show invited me to sit next to Charlie as millions of American viewers tuned in to witness Lauer ask the bombshell questions: Did Charlie have HIV? When did he know? Were others exposed? How was he coping? But Lauer also wanted an inside medical consultant to give straight answers to questions like, did Charlie have AIDS? What was his treatment? What was his prognosis?

Matt Lauer said it best near the beginning of the interview: This was blockbuster news, but also an important educational moment.

We live in a country with little if any sex education, and even less STD education! You can try to research HIV (or any of the other 30 sexually transmitted diseases) on the web, but good luck! Separating fact from internet fiction is next to impossible. Even the Centers for Disease Control site sometimes relies on out-of-date consensus statements.

Worldwide, five billion condoms are sold each year, but still, 1 million people get a new STD — *each and every day!* And then often pass that STD to loved ones, usually unknowingly. As a foot soldier on the frontlines in the STD battle, I feel it's important to fight these insidious threats to our well-being whenever possible.

Talking about HIV and Charlie's situation was a start. Little did I know that the *Today Show* appearance would set off a firestorm of indignant comments and shaming — not just about Charlie but about me as well.

I had witnessed shaming and racism before.

As the Los Angeles Raiders' team physician, hanging with players on road games, I witnessed racism for the first time: dismissive waitresses, boorish club doorman and belligerent "peace" officers who loathed African Americans.

Decades later, as the doctor for NBC's *The Biggest Loser*, leading 36 morbidly obese contestants through exercises on a stretch of Manhattan Beach, I witnessed fat shaming for the first time. As we ambled up from the wet ocean sand to the crowded strand sidewalk, I heard scores of weekend beachgoers derisively hoot and holler "fat ass!" and much, much worse.

Ten years later, I was by Charlie Sheen's side as he revealed his HIV positive status. Although much of the media was supportive, there were also hateful and ignorant posts. The vilest was *New York Post* writer Andrea Peyser, who in a giant headline the day after the announcement declared Mr. Sheen *"untouchable"* and me *"a repulsive 'helper doc.'"*

Excerpts from Peyser's article:

The put-away-wet actor revealed Tuesday that he has an enabler helping him procure women... for bareback fun: Dr. Robert Huizenga of Beverly Hills.

Sheen said he'd had condom-less sex after his diagnosis.

"But the two people I did it with were under the care of my doctor," he said.

Since when does a physician perch himself at a patient's bedside and toss out pointers about doing the deed without getting someone sick, or getting sued?

Only in Hollywood does a guy have a cheering section when he goes to bed with a loaded gun in his shorts...

While I had repeatedly witnessed HIV shaming over the past three decades, this was the first time I personally endured public HIV humiliation. No one likes it when their name is dragged through the mud in a national publication. It's especially exasperating when the media misinterpreted and misrepresented critical facts about HIV — specifically, how the *New York Post* took something incredibly positive (a game-changing medical protocol allowing safe condom-less sex with an HIV positive individual) and twisted it to make me the devil. What's that line? "No good deed goes unpunished."

I still remember re-reading the *New York Post* piece in my hotel room the morning after the *Today Show* interview. After a brief self-pity party, I vowed to combat the misinformation and the shaming.

I started to jot down misconceptions and outright lies about sexually transmitted diseases I'd read and heard just over the preceding few days.

This book is the result.

CHAPTER 3
The Announcement

It was an intense morning, even by *Today Show* standards.

Everything had happened at lightning speed. Just 48 hours prior, Charlie Sheen had decided to go public with his HIV diagnosis and had asked me to accompany him to discuss the medical nuances of his ordeal. The live, national TV interview didn't make me nervous. The facts were the facts. But I was beyond frantic when 30 minutes before airtime, the PR folks offhandedly asked me to write a medical statement to be mass-released during Charlie's appearance. It was a highly technical medical document that the press, thousands of HIV experts and millions of lay persons would read, and ultimately thoroughly dissect and interpret. I would ordinarily spend a whole week in the library writing and rewriting a document of that magnitude!

Suddenly, Matt Lauer popped into the green room and confidently shook Charlie's hand.

"Anything you want me to ask you?" Matt asked. His tailored suit pants seemed odd, literally skin tight, like a pair of spandex Nike running pants.

"No, I'm good," Charlie replied before Matt turned and quickly disappeared out of the green room door.

A minute later, we got our cue to head up to the set. Charlie, by nature unflappable, was counseled by his PR guy just as we stepped on the live *Today Show* set.

"You know how you always answer questions with your brilliant wit?" the PR agent asked.

"Yeah?"

"Don't do that this morning," he replied. "You've got to be dead serious."
Newsflash: Never give a comedic icon an anti-humor directive seconds prior to air time. Charlie gave him that you've-got-to-be-kidding-me look, but the last-second counsel mostly stuck. Charlie's speech was as deliberate as I've

ever seen. Matt, on the other hand, seemed edgy. I'm sure he did not want to lack empathy but was intent on asking tough questions. Still, he stumbled as he tiptoed through the emotional quagmire surrounding one of mankind's deadliest, most horrific medical epidemics.

The interview finished smoothly. But the aftermath – OMG! The maelstrom around sex and life-threatening STDs — no surprise. But the ignorance about STDs was a shock! Internet "experts" routinely spout misinformation, so tabloid "paparazzi" writers' hyperbolic half-truths accusing Sheen — and me — of unconscionably exposing his former female partners to deadly doses of HIV was not unexpected.

But the conventional print media? Big-city newspapers should be responsible about medical information critical to the public. Instead, some seem to have no idea about the true risk of contracting HIV and failed to fact-check. Here's a botched 2015 misquote from the *Boston Globe*.

> "Huizenga insisted that, given the reduced level of Sheen's virus, the chances that he has infected his partners are almost — but not entirely — negligible."
> "The chances of giving it are probably eight instances out of ten thousand," Huizenga said.
> "Even if Sheen isn't wearing protection?"
> "No protection, no nothing,' replied Huizenga."

Huh?!? This passage is rubbish. The statistic is garbage.

I never said that. The statistic I gave in the interview was very different.

"Eight instances out of ten thousand" is the chance an untreated HIV-positive male infects a female partner per episode of unprotected vaginal intercourse. Untreated does not apply here. Sheen was fully treated. I repeatedly called the *Globe* for a correction. No response.

Huh? What happened to reporters' holding accuracy sacrosanct? I can reluctantly understand why cost constraints might prevent beat writers from sending their first drafts to expert sources to confirm the veracity of scientific quotes, but in this case, I repeatedly contacted the newspaper afterward with the following correct quote.

> "Huizenga insisted that, given the undetectable level of Sheen's virus after anti-retroviral treatment (ART), and his partners' pre-exposure prophylaxis (PrEP), the chance he could infect his partners is essentially zero."
> "At most, the theoretical upper estimate of transmission is eight out of one hundred million after one contact—about the chance of being killed by lightning," Huizenga said.
> "Even if Sheen isn't wearing protection?"

"'No protection, no nothing,' replied Huizenga."

Why would the *Boston Globe* be so careless?
But *New York Post* columnist Andrea Peyser sunk lower. She mixed equal parts ignorance and intolerance in her article condemning — under any circumstance — the concept of "touching" an HIV-positive person, specifically Mr. Sheen. She editorialized about Mr. Sheen's statement that he had had sex without a condom with previous girlfriends.

"Charlie Sheen," Peyser wrote, "...goes to bed with a loaded gun in his shorts...Why would anyone touch him?"

Did Peyser do even one shred of research? Search the internet? Phone a knowledgeable Infectious Disease specialist? She certainly didn't bother to reach out to me for a comment.

She implied Mr. Sheen was going to kill his sexual partners ("(Sheen) goes to bed with a loaded gun in his shorts") and seemed to declare HIV persons are untouchables ("... why would anyone touch him?").

My reply: In terms of HIV risk, what's safer for a woman?

A. Having sex without a condom with a HIV-positive man (assuming the couple is treated by an HIV knowledgeable doctor)?

B. Having a one-night stand using condoms with a random guy from a local nightclub?

Answer: **A.**
I'll elaborate on this answer in Chapter Six.

CHAPTER 4
Human Immunodeficiency Virus (HIV): Back in a Time Machine

"When the history of AIDS and the global response is written, our most precious contribution may well be that, at a time of plague, we did not flee, we did not hide, we did not separate ourselves."

— Dr. Jonathan Mann (human rights advocate for HIV-positive individuals)

In 1980, the world was oblivious to HIV. Not even one case had been described.

Unbeknownst to me, I lived and worked that year at the ground zero of HIV, one of the most horrific epidemics in the history of mankind — a contagion so virulent that in three short decades it exploded from zero reported cases to 75 million potentially fatal infections in men, women and children alike.

I was a lowly medical resident, seeing uninsured walk-in patients at Cedars-Sinai Medical Center in Los Angeles. At that early stage of medical training, every sick patient's complaints are unfamiliar and tough to decipher. Almost always, with time and help from consultants, I'd figure out the diseases these folks had and with help from my handy spiral *Manual of Medical Therapeutics*, I'd eventually prescribe the right set of medications or lifestyle changes.

But just as my diagnostic confidence was growing, I began to see young, "healthy" patients who defied medical logic. They had complaints I couldn't figure out. One patient, a chef with non-stop fevers, was especially frustrating. He worked for a famous disease-phobic Hollywood producer who made his employees get their temperature taken at his front door before being allowed to report to work. My patient felt perfectly fine but his persistent low-grade temperatures had gotten him banned from his job for the last month. He came into the clinic for antibiotics and a back-to-work note. I examined him and found tender, enlarged neck lymph nodes. On his return visit a week later, I proudly presented him with my diagnosis: mononucleosis. His blood test results were classic. No treatment required. I confidently assured him he'd be fine in a month.

The chef dutifully returned in a month. I was disappointed to hear his fevers persisted and his neck nodes were larger. A new, more exhaustive lab panel revealed sky-high markers for cytomegalovirus — a more tenacious infection. Whew! I had him figured out after all. I told him no treatment was available, but he would kick the virus and heal in another four to six weeks.

A month later he returned with his male life partner. I was dismayed to hear not only had his fever not abated, he'd lost 10 pounds without trying and his lymph nodes were now gargantuan. An overwhelming sense of dread enveloped every inch of my slouched body. I was an idiot. Of course! These were classic "B" symptoms of Hodgkin's Disease. It was an aggressive lymphoma all along. I had whiffed on an obvious diagnosis! I scheduled him for an urgent open-neck-node biopsy. I bugged the 8th-floor lymphoma pathologist every painful self-critical day for the earliest hint of the results.

I still remember where I was standing when I got the pathologist's call. The chef's tissue showed benign inflammation. No fungus. No TB. And thank God no cancer!

I breathed a deep sigh of relief for my patient — and for me.

Now I was laser focused. I read every last page about fever of unknown origin and enlarging lymph nodes. Nothing matched up. Finally, an infectious disease buddy, Dr. Irv Posalski, who played second base on our aptly named *No Code Blue* doctor softball team, turned me onto Dr. Michael Gottlieb, a UCLA immunologist who was studying gay men with non-stop oddball infections and broken-down immune systems. OMG! The chef's condition fit Gottlieb's group to a T! Very frankly, my gaydar was never that great, so I wouldn't have figured out the gay part if not for meeting the life partner. In 1980, doctors didn't inquire into a patient's sexual orientation and I was no exception. It was rude and medically impertinent, right? I immediately sent my non-stop-fever chef crosstown for a consultation. To my amazement, just several months later, June 3, 1981, an official report in the

Centers for Disease Control *Morbidity Mortality Report* authored by Gottlieb and Posalski detailed five previously young, healthy, Los Angeles gay men with persistent fevers, unusual infections and immune system defects. This was the first ever written report of what would in short order become known as "AIDS" for Acquired Immune Deficiency Syndrome.

Immediately, the floodgates opened. Scores of doctors in what would soon be known as the four corners of AIDS — Los Angeles, San Francisco, New York City, and Miami — recognized more than 200 similarly perplexing patients. Kaposi's skin sarcoma, a dark red bruise-like lesion on the skin that got worse, not better (heretofore incredibly rare and seen only in geriatric Mediterranean men) was now routinely seen in young gay men in every hospital ward.

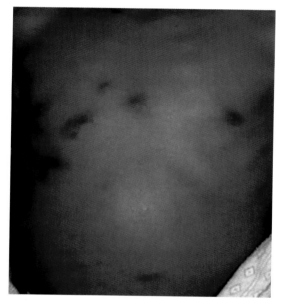

Half of the men with Kaposi's skin lesions were dead by year's end. The AIDS epidemic began its chilling upward explosion.

You think the incredibly rapid increase in these cases elicited a nationwide panic?

No. It yielded nothing more than a collective yawn. Several back-page stories appeared in the *New York Times*, but nobody sounded the alarms. It was regarded as someone else's problem.

It was just a "gay disease."

Figure 1 - Kaposi's skin sarcoma cancer, dark red bruise-like lesions

Attacking AIDS meant the gay lifestyle was put under the microscope. Was it something about oral and/or anal sex? Some immune-busting chemical? Or a ubiquitous street drug? I would ask patients about amyl nitrite poppers, the little yellow vials omnipresent on every exclusive LA and NYC disco floor. In fact, the constant mist behind the velvet ropes as you entered Club 54 was rumored to be amyl nitrate. Lots of doctors believed these chemicals damaged immune cells and were the villain. We continued to ask questions. Could a virus cause this syndrome? Cytomegalovirus caused fever, weight loss, big lymph nodes and might cripple the immune system. But a viral cause seemed unlikely. Could a virus trigger cancer? In 1980, most of my medical mentors felt the answer was no.

The gay community losses in Los Angeles began to mount. Day after day, patients were admitted to the Cedars Sinai wards with life-threatening conditions. A diagnostic test would have been nice, but it wasn't really needed. AIDS patients were gay, short of breath and rail-thin with apprehensive, sunken eyes. We blasted their infections and cancers with a potent array of drugs, but despite our efforts, after several admissions, the outcome was always the same. Death. Meanwhile, the media was busy with "more important" medical stories. For instance, in October 1982, all headlines for a solid month involved the seven deaths from cyanide-laced Tylenol. In stark contrast, there was only rare back-page coverage of the AIDS epidemic, now afflicting over 1 thousand Americans.

Just as the dread of this medical nightmare was permeating the gay community — two years after I first met the non-stop-fever chef — the other shoe dropped. Reports documented heterosexuals now succumbing to AIDS. They happened to be hemophiliacs who received regular infusions of blood clotting factors pooled from over a thousand donors. Immediately afterward, AIDS was reported in infants and heterosexual adults who had received ordinary blood transfusions. Then AIDS was confirmed in 34 heterosexual male and female Haitian migrants, and finally in female partners of male AIDS patients.

AIDS had been a rare, academically interesting disease — "someone else's" problem. Almost overnight, AIDS transformed into a disease anyone could get.

AIDS was no longer a "gay" disease.

AIDS had been a rare, academically interesting disease — "someone else's" problem. Almost overnight, AIDS transformed into a disease anyone could get.

AIDS was no longer a "gay" disease.

But America remained in denial. In early 1983, I saw firsthand just how deep that denial was. I had gotten an after-work job fact-checking medical stories for *The Today Show's* Dr. Art Ulene. He was adored by U.S. housewives and used his unique platform to cover medical topics from mundane flu outbreaks to cancer detection. I lucked out because he was a gynecologist and liked having internal medicine doctors like me do the background research on topics outside of his immediate comfort zone.

One afternoon, maybe during my sixth week of work, I had the single best idea of my life. I sat opposite Dr. Art Ulene, and passionately pitched my story idea:

America is in the middle of an epidemic that might soon rival the Black Plague. Hundreds and hundreds of gay men are dying. But this isn't a gay disease. It can be transmitted with vaginal sex! It can be transmitted with blood products and blood transfusions! More than 20 million people in the last two years have gotten transfusions! And they are having sex with their wives or husbands. What hidden iceberg are we cruising toward?

There is no test and no treatment. The only clues are that the AIDS agent:
- *is lethal to the immune system*
- *causes cancer*
- *is transferred via sex and blood transfusions*
- *is transferred when blood is filtered through miniscule pores (during the manufacture of blood clotting factors) so the AIDS agent is the size of a virus or smaller*

I ended by reminding him that nothing of significance had ever been revealed on national TV. We were going to break what potentially could be the medical story of the century on a morning TV show - and save lives too!

I sat bolt upright, expecting to be called a genius.
"Rob," he exhaled, "it's not my demographic."
"What?" I was in disbelief.
"My audience is middle American women. They are not interested in this story."

The next day I quit.

Thankfully, the world's premier virologists were not quitting. They had run through every clue and concluded only one entity fit the bill: *retro viruses.* Hypercompetitive Robert Gallo at the National Cancer Institute in Bethesda, Maryland and Luc Montagnier from the Pasteur Institute in Paris, France raced to solve the mystery, get bragging rights and along with Gottlieb (who was researching the exact HIV induced lymphocyte deficiency), claim an almost certain Nobel Prize.

On May 20, 1983, Luc Montagnier reported the discovery of a retrovirus named Lymphadenopathy Associated Virus (LAV) that he believed to be the cause of AIDS. Not every scientist agreed this was the true culprit, but suddenly AIDS was fully out of the closet.

At this point, mainstream America started to panic. When people panic, they make rash decisions. People with AIDS — and by extension, all gays — were treated as modern-day lepers.

AIDS patients were evicted from their apartments. Doctors who took care of AIDS patients were threatened with eviction by freaked-out landlords. Hemophiliac children were banned from schools. Police demanded special masks and gloves when dealing with possible infected criminals. Prison inmates revolted in fear as IV drug abuser cellmates started dying. Nurses quit rather than have to deal with AIDS patients. Funeral directors refused to embalm anyone with AIDS conditions on the death certificate. Subway riders wore gloves or took their chances with lurching trains and kept their hands off the rails.

In September 1983, the Center for Disease Control tried to calm the country's nerves by stating that AIDS could not be transferred by casual contact, food, water, air or environmental surfaces. But the medical basis for these claims was tenuous. A study of the first 2 thousand cases revealed about 90 percent fit the "4 H" mnemonic — homosexuals, Haitians, hemophiliacs/blood recipients or heroin (IV drug users) — or their sex partners. That left 10 percent who conceivably could have gotten it some other way. Poor sanitation? Kissing? Toilet seats? Contact with diarrhea or vomit? Mosquitoes?

Panic was surfacing big time in doctor lounges too.

Rumors spread that one of the original patients in Gottlieb's paper would supplement his income by donating blood. And that a premature baby given blood in our very own neonatal unit died of AIDS just several years post-transfusion. The rapidity of that death was unimaginable. We had never seen an infectious agent this dangerous. The CDC told us the AIDS virus was on par with hepatitis B. That was simultaneously insulting and laughable because Hep B was a walk in the park compared to AIDS. They recommended we gown, glove and goggle up when coming in contact with any "blood, excretions, secretions and body tissues" just in case this bug could cross intact skin or eye membranes or linger on clothes. That was too little too late. We'd already been exposed to the bodily fluids of scores of AIDS patients for years with no protection. Skin exposure? Come on, be real. Needle pricks? I'd gotten three or four sticks per year over the course of my medical training. Secretion exposure? Check. I'd taken full frontal vomit hits after difficult midnight intubations, not to mention exposure from mouth-to-mouth resuscitations.

We joked about the monks who had cared for bubonic plague victims. But we all knew that more monks died than any other segment of 14th-century society. Like the horrendous Black Death, the AIDS panic was causing otherwise intelligent people to murmur out loud *this was punishment from the heavens.* Sanctimonious hospital doctors even had an acronym ascribing the deities' purported opinion of a gay lifestyle. When yet another patient was admitted to the ward with the now all-too common constellation of fever, swollen lymph nodes, racking cough and dark bruise-like blotches — certain residents would mutter, "another WOG hit" (translated: another *Wrath of God* admission).

Most of my resident peers were not this callous, but we were emotionally and intellectually in over our heads. We were part realistic, part fatalistic and all in denial. I felt fine and pushed the possibilities into the back of my mind. Other doctors handled the fear differently. I'd call a surgical consult on an AIDS patient, only to hear some variant of this polite refusal, "Sorry, my wife is pregnant with our first child; I promised her I wouldn't take flagrant risks." Spoiler alert: Most of the time a baby bump never materialized.

Our hospital bosses were conspicuous by their silence. They never uttered a word. No acknowledgement of our 24/7 contagion fears. No risk-reduction classes, no staff psychotherapy, no family therapy for the significant other terrified at home.

It was every doctor for him or herself.

On April 23, 1984, Margaret Heckler, Secretary of the U.S. Department of Health and Human Services, amid much fanfare, announced that Robert Gallo had proved the retrovirus HTLV-III caused AIDS. She also announced a diagnostic blood test to identify the AIDS virus was right around the corner and predicted a vaccine against AIDS would be produced within two years.

In June 1984, Gallo and Montagnier held a joint press conference to announce that Montagnier's Lymphadenopathy Associated Virus (LAV) and Gallo's HTLV-III viruses are identical and the cause of AIDS. The virus name was changed to human immunodeficiency virus (HIV).

What follows is a brief summary of AIDS headlines for the next decades:

1985 – The CDC announced 10,000 Americans had AIDS, killing most within two years of diagnosis without a single documented recovery.

1985 – Conservative Surgeon General C. Everett Koop got the greenlight to craft the Reagan Administration's very first message to the American people. If anyone doesn't believe STDs are highly political, please reread the last sentence three or four times.

1985 – Belle Glade, Florida, an impoverished immigrant town, was revealed as having the world's highest density of HIV-positive persons. A disproportionately large percent were heterosexual men and women with none of the "4 H" risk factors. Were local mosquitoes indiscriminately transferring HIV?

Now No One Is Safe from AIDS screamed the headlines on the widely read July, 1985, installment of *Life* magazine which chronicled the Belle Glade epidemic. The cover showed a portrait of a wide-eyed young woman alongside pictures of a young father and mother holding a crying baby alongside a stiffly saluting American military officer.

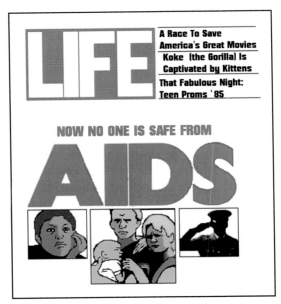

A Race To Save
America's Great Movies
Koke (the Gorilla) Is
Captivated by Kittens
That Fabulous Night:
Teen Proms '85

NOW NO ONE IS SAFE FROM

AIDS

Figure 2 - An artist's rendering of the Life Magazine *cover, 1985*

1985 – HIV blood test developed. Immediately, an American-French legal battle royale erupted over who had patent rights. Predictably, most of my high-risk patients refused to test. *"I don't want to know. There's nothing I can do. I'm already assuming I'm positive in terms of partners."* I, like other frontline doctors, was nervous about hospital exposures, but I wanted to know, so I did take the new HIV test.

1985 – Former presidential candidate Lyndon LaRouche introduced a ballot referendum in California stating employers could fire persons with AIDS and facilitate government-mandated "quarantines." Initially, polls suggested it could win. FYI: Isolation has no value unless a disease can be spread by casual contact.

1985 – Iconic actor Rock Hudson revealed he had AIDS and died shortly thereafter. He was a friend of Ronald Reagan, who many felt stonewalled meaningful government programs for fear of alienating his conservative political base. "The single most influential patient ever," said Michael Gottlieb, who was called in as Hudson's AIDS specialist. "His announcement, was the pivotal event in the country's consciousness of the HIV epidemic."

1986 – Surgeon General Koop released an explicit manifesto on how the AIDS virus is spread via shared blood products and vaginal, oral and anal intercourse — and how it is not spread, i.e. by casual touching or kissing.

1986 – CDC researchers in Belle Glade, Florida refuted the theory of mosquito transmission of AIDS. The unexpectedly high number of female and heterosexual males were traced to sex workers.

1986 – Lyndon LaRouche's California ballot referendum lost (71 percent to 29 percent) due in part to the opposition's "Stop the AIDS concentration camps" slogan.

1987 – Innovative additional HIV test (Western blot) was developed, which when combined with standard HIV test (ELISA) added accuracy.

1987 – Los Angeles Raiders became the first pro sports team to test for HIV. Some players had risk factors, and in the course of a season, players were frequently in contact with blood from other players. All players tested negative.

1987 – U.S. President Ronald Reagan and French Prime Minister Jacques Chirac called a truce in the patent wars by proclaiming Gallo and Montagnier "co-discoverers" of the virus and agreeing to split HIV testing patent royalties between the two countries.

1987 – Michael Gottlieb, potentially in line for a Nobel Peace Prize, was admonished by UCLA administrators for his frequent media appearances as "unbecoming to an academic" and finally denied tenure (professional advancement) at UCLA despite authoring more than 50 journal articles, including the classic first description of AIDS and the hallmark first description of HIV induced lymphocyte immune deficits.

1987 – First anti-HIV drug (AZT) was approved. Amazingly, approval only took two years between the drug identification in a lab and when it was available for doctors to prescribe — the fastest FDA approval of any drug. Gottlieb had a hand in its development.

1987 – Cedars-Sinai Hospital got sued for transfusing tainted blood from 1980 to 1985, but they prevailed in court. Cedars looked back at 700 babies they'd transfused in the neonatal unit in early '80s. At least 34 infants contracted HIV (four currently remain alive). Worldwide, a million individuals were HIV-infected with contaminated blood or blood products.

1991 – NBA superstar Magic Johnson revealed he was HIV positive. Magic got shingles. Shortly thereafter, a routine insurance exam revealed HIV. He was presumed to be early in the course of the disease and immediately began one of Dr. David Ho's controversial multidrug anti-retroviral cocktails.

1991 – Freddie Mercury, rock superstar, was diagnosed much later in the course of his disease and died.

1995 – Eazy-E, rap superstar, falsely believing his chronic cough is asthma, was admitted to Cedars where end-stage AIDS was diagnosed. He died one month later.

1996 – Multiple drug anti-retroviral cocktails became the standard of care. They were initiated later in the course of HIV infection when the immune system was noted to falter.

2008 – Nobel Prize in Physiology or Medicine was awarded to Montagnier for the discovery of HIV. Gallo and Gottlieb were left out.

Fast forward to 2011, literally *30 years* and *75 million* cases of HIV after I cared for the fever-of-unknown-origin chef.

Charlie Sheen walked into my Beverly Hills office complaining of sore throat, cough, joint pains and killer headaches. He'd started two weeks before with routine flu complaints. His voice doctor prescribed an antibiotic based on a positive throat culture but the throat pain never abated.

I got no clues from his physical exam. The odds favored a self-limiting viral reaction but out of an overabundance of caution, I ordered a bevy of infection tests. The infection panels, including an HIV test, returned perfectly normal, supporting my initial impression that this was indeed a self-limited benign viral "thing." But three days later, Day 17 from the start of his "flu," Charlie took a sudden turn for the worse. He got a stiff neck and his headache exploded, bursting from a 4 on the pain scale to a "12 out of 10."

His symptoms screamed meningitis. I had him rushed to the hospital for an urgent spinal tap and yet another plethora of esoteric body fluid infection tests. I was momentarily frozen when the results first flashed up on the hallway work station screen. The HIV test, just three days after being perfectly normal, was now positive!

There remained one sliver of hope: The "confirmatory" HIV Western blot test was normal. So, this could still possibly be a rare, three-in-a-thousand "false positive" HIV test result. There was also the 997/1000 probability this was a "seroconversion"— each one of his HIV tests flipping to abnormal as his immune system started producing telltale antibodies around three to four weeks after contracting HIV.

Day 23 the sliver of hope evaporated. The confirmatory Western blot had converted to positive as well. Next the viral load test done on day 19 returned positive — the number of HIV particles was through the roof — 4.4 million virions per cc of blood! There was now no question as to the correct diagnosis.

We immediately placed Charlie on four anti-retroviral drugs. We were full proponents of Dr. David Ho and his prescient mantra: Hit it hard. Hit it early. Mission accomplished. Charlie's HIV viral blood levels promptly plummeted to zero over the next several months and stayed there.

Given the fact that treatment consistently suppressed viral quantities to undetectable levels (typical of properly treated individuals), Charlie's HIV only minimally — if at all — affects his predicted life expectancy. I'm much more concerned about his cigarette intake.

The Charlie Sheen Effect:

When Charlie decided to come forward, I felt he would save many more lives with his honest revelation than I could ever have aspired to as a doctor. Still, I was blown away by the "Charlie Sheen Effect," elucidated in two medical journal articles documenting the lasting benefits of his *Today Show* announcement — ironically 35 years and 35 million HIV deaths after my *Today Show* HIV story pitch was summarily rejected as not newsworthy to middle American women — or anyone else!!!

Post announcement, there was a 540 percent increase in HIV-related internet searches. There was a doubling of at-home HIV test sales for a month.

These increases were astounding: seven times larger than that associated with World AIDS Day, the largest and longest-running HIV prevention awareness event.

"The public health system is top-down, and informational messages come mainly from experts. We forgot to listen to the public, and this is what the public is engaging on," explained study co-author Eric Leas. "It's an empowering message. The truth is that you can make a difference by just speaking out. We all hear talk is cheap. That's not true."

"I had patients come in and ask me questions," said Dr. Barron Lerner, a professor of medicine at NYU and an expert on the national health impact of famous patients. "Some of them assume he must have used drugs or had unprotected sex with a man. I'm like, you know, that's not necessarily the case at all."

Study co-author, Dr. JP Allem, commented on the transference of sympathy: "Our findings build on earlier studies that suggest empathy is easier to motivate in others when the empathy is targeted toward an individual versus a group. It is easy to imagine that a single individual, like Sheen, disclosing his HIV status may be more compelling and motivating for people than an unnamed mass of individuals or lectures from public health leaders."

Fact is, the public is listening, but now, there is a new learning dynamic — "the Charlie Sheen Effect." Viral social media health stories provide an opportune teaching moment, resonating with the public more than "traditional" medical messaging from the surgeon General or local public health officials.

CHAPTER 5
HIV: Today's Facts and Falsehoods

How many persons get new infections each year (HIV incidence)?

In 2017, 38,000 new HIV diagnosis were made in the U.S. New cases due to childbirth and breastfeeding cases are common worldwide but rare (128 cases) in the U.S.

HIV, an absolute terror in the '80s and '90s, today mostly elicits complacency. But make no mistake: despite gigantic advances in diagnosis and treatment, and the gradual decrease in new cases, HIV is still a disease to be reckoned with — worldwide, more than 2 million people still catch HIV each year. Half of those new cases will be women and children.

How many persons are currently infected (HIV prevalence)?

In the United States, 1.1 million people are currently HIV positive. Fifty-five percent of HIV-positive Americans are gay or bisexual men, 22 percent are heterosexual men and 23 percent are women.

Worldwide, 37 million people are currently HIV positive.

Death rates have plummeted recently, but still there were 6,700 American deaths directly attributable to HIV/AIDS in 2017.

How do I get HIV?

HIV is a sexually transmitted disease (STD). It can be transmitted via vaginal or anal intercourse. HIV is also spread via tainted blood (transfusions, shared needles, accidental needle sticks or transplant tissue) and via vaginal childbirth and breastfeeding.

Contagiousness is directly related to:
- the number of viral particles in the blood, semen, vaginal or rectal secretions
- the HIV-positive person's awareness. Seventeen percent of the 1.1 million Americans with the infection are unaware they have it
- the HIV infection stage
- the integrity of the oral, vaginal and rectal mucous membranes
- the presence of cuts, scrapes or infections (i.e. other STDs) which can damage the integrity of mucous membranes

You cannot get HIV from:
- causal contact
- kissing
- hugging
- shaking hands
- sharing personal objects, food or water
- mosquitoes

What Are the First Warning Signs of HIV?

Several weeks after the initial HIV infection, most but not all persons experience a flu-like illness typically including one or more of these symptoms: fever, chills, rash, night sweats, muscle aches, sore throat, fatigue, headaches, swollen lymph nodes and/or mouth ulcers.

There is no "smoking gun" complaint. Still a light bulb should go off if even an "ordinary" flu occurs two to six weeks after a high risk sexual hook-up.

HIV: What happens if you don't treat

HIV reproduces rapidly after the initial infection. During the first months, extremely high numbers of viral particles in the millions per cubic centimeter (one teaspoon equals five cubic centimeters) course through the blood. In relatively short order, the body's immune system fights back and lowers, but cannot eliminate, the virus.

For the next five to 10 years, it's a raging stalemate between the immune system and the virus. HIV viral loads drop from the 3 - 4 million to the 50,000 particles per cc range — levels low enough to often keep infected persons feeling healthy. Not surprisingly, many individuals live through this "silent stage" never thinking to get tested.

Finally, the body's defenses are overrun. The viral load (the number of replicating viruses per cc of blood) cruises upward as the wheels of the immune system wobble and then fall off. "AIDS" begins, manifested by fevers, diffuse enlarged lymph nodes and weight loss (like my non-stop-fever chef) followed by continuous perilous infections (especially tuberculosis) and cancers (especially lymphomas and Kaposi's sarcoma (Figure 1), which a healthy immune system could easily swat away.

Despite state-of-the-art antibiotic and anticancer treatments, if no specific anti-HIV therapy is initiated, death is inevitable two to three years after the onset of AIDS.

How is HIV diagnosed?

The first step in diagnosing HIV is an index of suspicion. Individuals engaging in certain high-risk activities — men who have sex with men (MSM), sex workers (exchanging money, drugs or presents for sex), multiple heterosexual partners, IV drug use and blood exposure — raise the suspicion flag. Individuals at very low risk, i.e. pregnant women and their partners, also should raise the suspicion flag, not because of high sexual or blood exposure risk, but because missing even one case of preventable mother-to-child transmission is unacceptable.

The second step is testing everyone with an index of suspicion every three to six months. Unhappily, studies show MSM test on average less than once a year and heterosexuals at high risk test only about every other year. Fortunately, HIV tests are extremely accurate. In the U.S., when the standard ELISA HIV antibody test says you are negative, you are truly HIV free 99.7 percent of the time! In other words, there is only an exceedingly small three-in-a-thousand percent chance of a wrong result.

The HIV "window" period throws a wrench into test interpretation. The usual HIV screening test (ELISSA antibody test) — remains negative for approximately four weeks after the start of a new infection because it takes a while for the body's immune system to produce measurable antibodies. In rare cases, the body's immune system responds even slower, prolonging the window period (the period of true infection but normal blood screening tests) to between three and six months in three percent of cases.

If the index of suspicion is high, we utilize a more accurate but also more expensive test — a RNA (ribonucleic acid) test — to shrink the "window period" down to 10-14 days after HIV infection. As you can imagine, blood banks add those RNA tests routinely to assure the safety of our blood supply. Some porn studios have also adopted this aggressive testing! They require adult film stars to test for HIV RNA every two weeks. Too bad they don't require testing for many other much more common STDs.

How is the accuracy of the confidential, convenient and affordable home tests? Very good — though not as good as the HIV RNA test. Persons with very recent infections face a 1-in-12 chance of not being detected (i.e. the test returns normal but the individual is really positive for HIV). Given the gravity of HIV, at-home testing should be used only to detect an infection at least three months old. To be 100 percent sure, after an initial negative test, repeat a home test 3 months later.

Mandatory testing by medical or government authorities is a bad idea. Not only does it infringe on human rights, it tends to be counterproductive by scaring high-risk persons "underground." Requiring hospitals or institutions like jails or prisons to offer everyone free and voluntary testing is a good compromise, which makes testing readily available without coercing anyone to be tested.

Is HIV curable?

No. Not yet.

Is HIV Treatable?

Yes. 100 percent.

HIV is treatable at all stages of the disease, but the earlier treatment begins, the better the outcome.

Who needs treatment? All HIV-positive children, adolescents and adults, including all pregnant and breastfeeding women, beginning immediately after diagnosis and continued for life.

HIV replicates in the body at breakneck speed: Millions and millions of viruses per cc course through the bloodstream just two weeks after infection. Anti-retroviral therapy (ART) neutralizes this replication frenzy, clearing the blood of detectable virus in about three months. Consequently, the immune system stays intact. AIDS, the result of our immune system's battling continual waves of reproducing HIV particles, never gets a chance to rear its ugly head. Instead of a death sentence — like I repeatedly gave in the 1980s — HIV-positive patients can now look forward to a near normal life expectancy. That drastic prognostic turnaround, in a mere two decades, is the most momentous medical advance of our lifetime.

**Instead of a death sentence — like I repeatedly
gave in the 1980s — HIV-positive patients can
now look forward to a near normal life expectancy.
That drastic prognostic turnaround, in a mere two decades,
is the most momentous medical advance of our lifetime.**

ART has been effective since the mid-1990s, as evidenced by Magic Johnson's health throughout the last three decades, but these earlier treatments had many liver, GI, skin, and metabolic side effects. Today, ART options exist with minimal side effects. (Nothing has zero side effects — not even aspirin or Tylenol!)

The first anti-HIV drug, AZT, was approved in 1987 but it never panned out. There were a slew of side effects and the HIV virus managed to quickly mutate in a manner making new strains resistant, an emotional saga revisited in *Dallas Buyers Club*. Other anti-HIV drugs were subsequently released that also nailed HIV in a test tube but disappointed in real life. Then, like the calvary riding in wearing white Stetsons, a new wave of brilliant docs cracked the resistance problem. Just as Magic Johnson was standing behind the Forum podium addressing a stunned nation, Dr. David Ho, my classmate at Harvard and my co-Chief Resident at Cedars-Sinai Hospital during the dark days of HIV, was formulating his *Hit It Hard, Hit It Early* poly-drug HIV attack. Using his math background, he calculated, based on HIV's astronomically high mutation rate, just how many simultaneous anti-virals it was going to take to prevent the HIV virus from changing just enough to repeatedly develop resistance.

He directed Magic Johnson's care, appeared on the cover of TIME magazine and in the process championed life-saving HIV drug cocktails.

One size does not fit all when it comes to anti-HIV treatment. Cocktails of three to five drugs (ART) are individually tailored based on the following factors:

a. **Potency.** Nowadays, most ART is potent, so this requirement is no longer the principal driver in personalized ART cocktails. Still, about one in six people on their first HIV treatment regimen either never reach an undetectable viral load or their treatment stops working in the first year or two. By the second or third regimen however, essentially everyone taking their ART pills as directed reduces viral load to undetectable (i.e. fewer than 20 to 40 virions per cc of blood).

b. **Ease of administration.** It's tough remembering handfuls of pills multiple times per day. Recently, some ART cocktails have been combined into just one daily pill.

c. **Safety and side effects:** This is still a big hurdle. Past anti-retro viral therapy was life-giving but frequently had nasty side effects. Even now, some "well tolerated" modern ART has nagging gut or low energy side effects. Hopefully, next-generation ART will solve this problem.

d. **Cost.** No matter the specific ART chosen, cost is the elephant in the room. Footing the monthly bill of ART is problematic in the U.S. without any coherent national health coverage. In many of the impoverished countries that bear the brunt of this relentless disease, medication is provided by U.S. foreign aid and distributed at no cost by the local government through bipartisan programs initiated by George W. Bush. Still, even with the generosity of the American people and contributions by local governments, over half of HIV positive persons in Africa are undiagnosed and untreated – something we must urgently change.

What are my chances of catching HIV?

Outside of the major causes — multiple sex partners, lack of condom use, lack of PrEP use and intravenous drug use — your chance of catching HIV depends on a host of other factors including the presence of other STD(s) you might have, the number of undiagnosed HIV infected persons with whom you have sex (i.e. higher risk in urban areas, among men who have sex with men and in the Southeast U.S.) and your overall health.

If you do have blood exposure or sex with an untreated HIV positive individual, your risk of contracting HIV is:

Risk Blood Exposure:
- HIV-positive blood transfusion 9,300 per 10,000 exposures (93%)
- Needle sharing with IV drug use 63 per 10,000 exposures (0.63%)
- Needle stick hospital accident 23 per 10,000 exposures (0.23%)
- Red Cross blood transfusion 1 in 2,500,000 exposures (0.00004%)

Risk Maternal Exposure:
- Vaginal delivery 2,500 per 10,000 exposures (25%)
- Breast feeding 1,000 per 10,000 exposures (10%)

Risk Sexual Exposure:
- Anal sex
  Receptive (bottom) 138 per 10,000 exposures (1.4%)
  Insertive (top) 11 per 10,000 exposures (0.11%)
- Vaginal sex
  Infected male 8 per 10,000 exposures (0.08%)
  Infected female 4 per 10,000 exposures (0.04%)
- Oral sex 1 per 10,000 or lower
- Deep French kissing with oral sores very low risk
- Biting through skin very low risk

No Risk
- Lip kissing
- Saliva or tear exposure
- Hugging, shaking hands

- Sharing food or water with common silverware/dishes/glasses
- Public toilet seat
- Coughing or sneezing

If you have intimate sexual contact with a fully treated HIV-positive individual (viral load undetected for more than six months), your risk of contracting HIV is:

Zero!

If you have intimate sexual contact with a fully treated HIV-positive individual (viral load undetected for more than six months), your risk of contracting HIV is:

Zero!

Too good to be true, right? That was my first thought too when I read the early research showing heterosexual HIV-infected patients with full viral suppression on successful ART did not infect partners. This quickly became more than just idle curiosity when Charlie Sheen and his then-girlfriend came to my office to discuss having a baby. I cobbled together a group of HIV experts and they concurred: HIV did not appear to infect partners of well-treated heterosexual HIV-infected persons. But given the limited numbers of patients in the initial studies five years ago, there still was the chance that larger future studies might show a one-in-a-million risk. Given the grave consequence of being wrong, we elected to have the woman simultaneously take anti-retrovirals as "pre-exposure prophylaxis" (PrEP) — at that early date a brand-new drug that when taken daily prevented HIV-negative persons from acquiring HIV.

If Charlie and his ex-partner approached me today with the same question, HIV specialists are so confident there is no risk of transmission when a person is fully treated, they no longer recommend PrEP for partners of patients with well treated HIV infection — or any other preventative, except for condoms to prevent other STDs.

How can I prevent contracting HIV?

a. Awareness is prevention
Persons oblivious of their HIV infection (or any other STD for that matter) unknowingly cause a disproportionate amount of new cases. Worldwide, up to 40 percent of HIV-positive individuals are unaware of their infection. In the U.S., about 17 percent are unaware of their HIV-positive status (25 percent in Louisiana).

We can do better.

Start by making HIV testing universally available ... and free. Then reach out to "at-risk" persons: MSM, heterosexuals with new partners, IV drug users and pregnant women. A pregnant woman is not technically "high risk," but missing a rare HIV case that would cause lifelong consequences, in my mind, is not an option. I never want to revisit what I witnessed in pediatric patients in the 1980s.

In America, troubling HIV facts remain:
- 660,000 MSM and bisexual American men are currently HIV positive - 15 percent of all MSM.
- 100,000 MSM and bisexual men are unaware of their HIV diagnosis - 2 to 3 percent of all MSM and bisexual men. We know this by studies of representative samples of MSM and bisexual men.
- 264,000 heterosexual men are HIV positive - 0.5 percent of sexually active "single" heterosexual men. About 50,000 heterosexual men are unaware of their HIV status.
- 276,000 "single" heterosexual women are currently HIV positive - 0.5 percent of sexually active "single" heterosexual women. About 50,000 heterosexual women are unaware of their HIV status.

b. Treatment is prevention
We now have the potential to diagnose and treat every HIV-infected person. Anti-retroviral therapy (ART) can suppress HIV so effectively that progression to deadly AIDS should be a thing of the past. But optimal ART does something else I never could have imagined.

ART can prevent HIV transmission.

And this is the headline news: ART prevents transmission of HIV in previously unthinkable settings — even when an HIV-positive man has vaginal intercourse without a condom with an uninfected woman. Just a few years ago, this was a felony punishable by jail time.

More unlikely still? Multiple studies now suggest ART also prevents HIV transmission during anal intercourse, a sexual practice 17-times riskier than vaginal intercourse.

Starting 10 years ago, there were enticing hints this was true, but until a recent European study, there weren't enough cases to calculate transmission rates from treated HIV-positive persons during high-risk sex. The European study evaluated 1,228 couples (one partner was HIV positive and on ART for six or more months, the other partner was HIV negative) who were having sex more than 40 times a year — with no condoms! Frankly, this study could not have been done in the U.S. due to the heightened HIV stigma. The existence of this many couples freely having sex without condoms in the face of diagnosed HIV is shocking to most Americans.

Bottom line: The 888 heterosexual and 340 MSM couples had 44,000 episodes of oral, vaginal and anal sex without condoms. The results? There was not one single transmitted case of HIV.

Not one case!

Without treatment, 50 to 100 new cases of HIV would have been expected!

Attention! HIV-discordant couples (one fully treated HIV positive, one negative individual) contemplating condom-less sex — these points are non-negotiable:

- The HIV-positive person must be maniacal about taking the ART as directed. Just a week off can result in rapidly rising viral loads.
- Viral load tests need to be done regularly to confirm that levels remain undetectable.
- The viral load needs to be completely suppressed for six or more months.
- Both partners need to be monitored for drug abuse and infections, including STDs, which can, in untreated HIV-positive individuals, increase HIV transmission. Surprisingly, however, in the above-noted European study, there was not a single HIV transmission even though many people had STDs.
- Always inform your partner if you are HIV positive. There are still states that make non-disclosure of HIV a felony, even when the chance of transmitting HIV is zero!

Even this impressive European study and several parallel research papers do not categorically prove that an optimally treated HIV positive person will *never* transmit HIV. It means that, at worse, transmission is extremely unlikely and at best it will never happen.

That is similar to U.S. Surgeon General Dr. Koop's declaration in his celebrated 1986 pamphlet to the American public at the peak of AIDS hysteria that *"HIV cannot be transmitted by kissing."*

This statement has never been proven, but as each decade passes without someone catching HIV via kissing, the veracity of the statement becomes more and more certain. Now 30 years later, with a massive amount of experience showing zero HIV transmission via kissing, the accuracy of the late Dr. Koop's statement is finally unquestioned.

Make no mistake though. There is far more evidence today supporting zero vaginal transmission in discordant couples with the HIV-infected partner fully treated in the above no-condom scenario than there was of zero saliva transmission in 1986 when Dr. Koop made his famous declaration.

**Andrea Peyser, please inform your NY Post readers
that fully treated HIV-positive individuals are not "infectious."
They do not carry a "loaded gun" in their shorts.**

---

c. Prophylaxis is prevention
The HIV "Pill" – *PrEP*
The first oral birth control pill was approved by the FDA on May 5, 1960. Within a few short years, the "pill" gained widespread acceptance, disconnecting sex — for the first time in human history — the act of unprotected, skin-on-skin sex from procreation. Centuries-old "immutable" interpersonal relationship patterns quickly changed. Out-of-marriage sex became "accepted," not some slutty back alley faux-pas. Then in quick succession came the tolerance of abortion, nudity and gay lifestyles — even to Main Street middle-class, middle-aged, middle-America.

In 2012, to little fanfare, the FDA approved another game changer: an "HIV prevention pill" called pre-exposure prophylaxis (PrEP). It has the potential to disconnect — for the first time since the devastating AIDS epidemic began — the sex act from the risk of HIV transmission, even without the use of a condom. By the end of 2017, 125,000 Americans were taking PrEP, a number that will almost certainly increase in the future as even today, the majority of doctors have either not heard of or have no idea how to prescribe this treatment.

PrEP is a combination of two anti-HIV drugs — trade name Truvada. If taken every day by an "at risk" HIV negative person — i.e. sexually active men who have sex with men (MSM), partners of a heterosexual HIV infected person, sex workers, IV drug users or heterosexual persons with high risk partners — it lowers the risk of getting HIV by 99 plus percent. The pill must be taken daily without fail and takes at least one week to be fully effective. By way of comparison, birth control pills (BCPs) also lower pregnancy risk by 99 percent and need to be taken daily without fail.

Today, six years after approval, PrEP's effects are reverberating through high-risk HIV populations, especially the MSM community. When I first began prescribing PrEP in 2013, I was petrified. For the last four decades, I had militantly warned my gay and all other high-risk patients to always use condoms or risk certain HIV. Now, approving condom-less sex with an HIV positive person? It sounded like heresy!

Understandably, this sudden turnabout — the fact PrEP appears to lower the risk of HIV more effectively than condoms (like birth control pills reduce unwanted pregnancies more effectively than condoms)—has shaken many preconceived notions and raised many new concerns.

Oh, Andrea, one more thing.

Doctors who prescribe effective anti-retroviral cocktails to HIV positive persons — and when indicated PrEP to uninfected partners — are not "enablers" of dangerous sex. They are conscientious care givers.

Does PrEP really work as well as advertised? I don't want to get HIV!

In real-world settings, PrEP isn't perfect, but it's damn close! There is no evidence supporting worries that if individuals forget an occasional pill they will get HIV. Only three cases of PrEP failure have been documented worldwide out of the hundreds of thousands of persons, mostly MSM, currently on this preventative pill. Of the three cases of PrEP failure, two were due to acquiring a rare HIV strain resistant to PrEP, the third got the run-of–the-mill HIV strain but had an unusually large amount of risky exposure: anal intercourse with hundreds of different partners over an eight-month period.

So, in real world use, the 99 plus percent HIV transmission-reduction claim appears right on target.

Does PrEP have side effects?

Truvada has an excellent safely record. Transient headaches and appetite loss can occasionally occur and there is a low risk of reversible kidney disease and mild lowering of bone mineral density (inconsequential to all but those with severe osteoporosis). The biggest negative is cost and the inconvenience of having to follow-up with the prescribing doctor every three months (these follow up visits are necessary to make sure no one on PrEP is positive for HIV or any other STD).

With the HIV risk off the table, will individuals have more sex?

Yes. It's fair to look at the experience of heterosexuals with the advent of birth control pills (BCPs) and not be surprised. With lower risk, people have more sex. Freedom to express one's sexuality — as in the '60s sexual revolution — is good news. PrEP would be expected to increase quality of life and removes the fear from an everyday, wonderful, healthy activity-sex.

The downside? Cost (thousands per month) and STDs. Condom-less sex inevitably translates to more STDs. Already clinics caring for large numbers of PrEP patients are reporting up to twenty-fold increases in syphilis, gonorrhea and chlamydia cases.

Can MSM, sex workers and heterosexual folks in high-risk Sub-Saharan countries on PrEP now feel free to have sex without condoms?

At-risk individuals have to decide if a greater than 99 plus percent risk reduction is good enough. Let me eliminate one common misunderstanding. I said before that having sex without a condom was fully safe if your partner was a fully treated HIV-positive person on ART. Above I said that if you are at risk of having sex without a condom with an untreated HIV person, then PrEP lowers that risk by 99 plus percent.

In terms of HIV transmission, all agree it's safer to have oral, vaginal or anal sex without a condom on PrEP (99-plus percent protection) than sex off PrEP with a condom (80 percent protection). By way of comparison, look back at the '60s: Couples on birth control pills with a 99 percent less chance of pregnancy overwhelmingly ditched condoms.

In 2012, when I advised discordant couples wanting to get pregnant, I relied on ART (HIV positive partner) plus PrEP (uninfected partner). Now, with studies showing effective ART prevents transmission, is the use of PrEP redundant?

The majority of HIV experts agree that the "added protection" of PrEP in this situation is unnecessary.

Who should be on PrEP?

PrEP is for those with a one percent per year or more chance of catching HIV. Potentially 500,000 to 1,000,000 Americans meet this criterion, mainly MSM, heterosexuals in ongoing relationships with an inadequately treated partner or those with high risk partners like sex workers, IV drug users or sexually active adolescents and young adults in countries with a high burden of HIV infection.

Personally, if I had between a one-in-a-hundred and one-in-a-thousand chance of contracting HIV, I would use PrEP. But unless I had a knowledgeable doctor (in 2016, only one in three primary care physicians had even heard of PrEP) and health insurance to pay the cost, I'd be out of luck.

"HIV Morning After Pill" – PEP
The HIV morning-after pill, called post-exposure prophylaxis (PEP), is an emergency 28-day regimen to be taken after HIV exposure: either sexual, (i.e. broken condom,

"forgetting" to use condom in the heat of the moment), accidental needle sticks (or shared needles) or blood spray to the eye or mouth. PEP is Truvada plus one more anti-HIV drug for added potency and must be started within two to three days of exposure — understandably the earlier the better.

Patients who repeatedly seek PEP should be considered for PrEP, as daily PrEP may be more protective than repeated episodes of PEP.

d. Protection is prevention: Condoms
Latex (or polyurethane) male or female condoms for decades were the gold standard for HIV and STD prevention. Condoms can hold water or even air (they make great balloons), so they can easily hold or block sperm, bacteria and even miniscule viruses. But let's be real. If people really used condoms as much as they should, would we have 1 million new STD infections and 6,000 new HIV infections globally — *each and every day?*

Let's be real.

If people really used condoms as much as they should, would we have 1 million new STD infections and 6,000 new HIV infections globally — each and every day?

Condoms are readily available. They're inexpensive (if you buy in bulk). They're easily transported (but don't leave in the glove compartment because heat can damage condoms). They have no side effects (except rarely latex allergy). Five billion are sold each year. They seem simple to use (once you figure out which side is up). They work great (if used properly). (See video on how to use a male condom by Planned Parenthood).

In real world experience, standard latex condoms are often used improperly… and infrequently. In America, only 50 percent of sexually active teens reported using condoms the last time they had sex, and the use only goes down as age increases. Increased STDs are not the only consequence. About 750,000 American teens get pregnant each year, 80 percent unplanned. By way of comparison, last year, 6.0 million American women got pregnant with 3.8 million live births, 1 million miscarriages and 1.1 million abortions.

Why the resistance to public health officials' pleas to use condoms?

1. The PC version: lack of education. The real reason: Sex is often less sexy. It may be less pleasurable; some condom types can deaden tactile stimulation.

2. Inability to get or maintain erections due to prolonged foreplay stoppage, condom neck pressure, or between-the-ears difficulties related to flashbacks of prior failed attempts.

3. Occasionally latex allergy (rash/itchiness) in either partner.

4. Partial brain death immediately prior to sex, which means available condoms remain unused.

5. Rubber smell/taste is a turn off.

6. Standard condoms are not a good man-junk look. They make the penis look like a small-town bank robber with an overstretched nylon face mask.

Solutions?

Lelo's Hex condom:
For those with problems with breakage, slippage, foreplay stoppage and tactile sensation diminution: Try a new easier-to-apply, one-half thinner, more natural, stronger, better-gripping condom.

Non-latex condoms:
For the occasional individual with latex allergies.

Lambskin:
Sorry, this is not the solution. Lambskin is claimed to be the closest thing to bareback and they're biodegradable (I cringe when yet another latex condom washes up on our California beaches), but here's the deal-breaker. Lambskin pore size, though small enough to block sperm, is too large to block viruses. It cannot prevent HIV, herpes or HPV transmission. Essentially, it's the equivalent of female birth control pills: a great contraceptive but no help with STD prevention.

If one looks at the 25 million STDs Americans catch each year, condoms if universally used can prevent less than 60 percent of new STDs! Condoms lower the risk of transmission of HPV, syphilis and herpes by only 50 percent because these infections can be transmitted via genital skin not covered by the condom. Clearly, condoms are important but other preventive strategies have to be used.

Perhaps, with less breakage and better grip, the new Lelo Hex technology can prevent an extra million or more STDs. Thankfully we have other extremely effective anti-STD approaches — which when used in parallel with condoms can further lower — or theoretically — eliminate STDs!

		New Infections/Yr.	Condom Effectiveness	If 100% Condom Use - Potential Drop of Infetions
NUMBER OF NEW STD INFECTIONS UNIVERSAL CONDOM USE MIGHT PREVENT IN THE U.S.				
Human Papilloma Virus (HPV)		14,000,000	50%	7,000,000
Herpes Simplex Virus (adult onset)		3,000,000		
HSV1 - oral	400,000		0%	0
HSV1 - genital	1,200,000		50%	600,000
HSV2 - genital	1,400,000		50%	700,000
Chlamydia		2,900,000	80%	2,320,000
Mycoplasma		2,800,000	80%	2,240,000
Trichomonas		1,100,000	80%	880,000
Gonorrhea		820,000	80%	656,000
Pubic Lice		120,000	0%	0
Syphilis		88,000	50%	44,000
Hepatitis		50,000		
Hep C	31,000		80%	24,800
Hep B	19,100		80%	15,280
Human Immunodeficiency Virus (HIV)		38,400	80%	30,720
TOTAL NUMBER NEW STD CASES (U.S.)		**24,916,400**		
Number of new STD cases condoms might prevent				**14,510,800**
Percent of new STD cases condoms might prevent				**58%**

Table 4

Condoms work well – but they may only be able to prevent 60% of new STDs

e. Talking Is Prevention

1. If you don't ask, your partner may be far less likely to tell.

2. If you do ask, don't assume the answer is truthful.

3. Inform your partner of any STDs you have, including HIV, even though now HIV transmission can be entirely prevented, unlike HPV and herpes where under the best of circumstances we have only partial prevention.

4. After sex, please discuss why many states (not California) still have laws making non-disclosure of HIV a felony even though stiff penalties may convince some to go underground and not test, paradoxically increasing HIV transmission.

5. Also talking is a good way to open the dialogue about condoms. How she or he likes to use a condom? Problems or concerns with condom use? It is always harder for a woman to bring up condom use with a man. It's a man thing after all. I advise my female patients to tell their male partners that they enjoy sex more with a condom. That condoms make her feel free, worry less

and help her orgasm more fully because she's not concerned about becoming pregnant or catching something.

And with a condom - no arguments about who has to sleep on the wet spot!

Always have condoms bedside. Bring condoms with you on trips. Be optimistic and bring a bunch! Women and men should both be responsible for having condoms available. Nothing is sexier than a woman (or male partner) bringing out a condom and lustily placing it on a man's penis. Many sex workers know how to put a condom on a penis by using just their mouth! Something to practice.

f. Planning is prevention
Male circumcision is a lesser known form of HIV protection, surprisingly lowering the risk in heterosexual men by 65 percent.

Lastly, in terms of addressing bloodborne HIV transmission, harm-reduction programs for injecting drug users (furnishing sterile injecting equipment, including needles, syringes and safe injection rooms) although counterintuitive, turn out to be beneficial.

In summary, have a comprehensive protection plan firmly in hand before you touch anything else.

Human Immunodeficiency Virus (HIV) Summary:

Incubation Period:
2 weeks to 2 months

Initial symptoms:
About 50% get flu-like illness, rash, sore throat, fever

What happens if no treatment:
Debilitating immunosuppression leading to AIDS 5 - 10 years after infection and death 2 - 3 years after onset AIDS. (AIDS = the onset of unexplained weight loss, fever, enlarged lymph nodes, rare infections and cancers)

Source of HIV infection:
- Blood, sperm (cum), pre-cum, rectal or vaginal secretions, breast milk
- Not spread by kissing or household contact (showers, toilet seats, towels)

Curable?
No

Treatable?
Yes, various anti-retroviral cocktails (ART's), normal or near normal life-expectancy

Prevention (risk reduction):
- monogamy (100%) with HIV uninfected partner
- optimal medication use by HIV positive persons (99 - 100%)
- optimal pre-exposure prophylaxis (PrEP) (daily meds used before high risk sex) (99%+)
- optimal post exposure prophylaxis (PEP) (28-day medication regimen taken after unprotected high risk sex) (90%+)
- condoms (80 - 85%)
- circumcision (65%)
- detection and treatment of another co-existing STD (up to 30%)

Incidence (new U.S. cases/year):
39,000

Total U.S. cases:
1,100,000

Infectivity (single contact with untreated patient or HIV tainted blood):

Very High
- Blood Transfusion: 93% risk transmission from HIV positive blood
- Vaginal Delivery: 25% risk transmission from untreated HIV positive mother
- Breast Feeding: 10% risk transmission from untreated HIV positive mother

High
- Anal sex: Receptive (bottom) - 1.4% risk transmission from untreated HIV positive partner

  Insertive (top) - 0.1% risk transmission from untreated HIV positive partner

- Needle sharing with drug use: 0.6% risk transmission from untreated HIV positive partner

- Needle stick, hospital accident: 0.23% risk transmission from untreated HIV positive source

- Vaginal sex: Infected male - 0.08% risk transmission (4% year if weekly sex)

  Infected female - 0.04% risk transmission (2% year if weekly sex)

Low
- Oral Sex: Receptive - Very low: about 5 well-documented cases

  Insertive - negligible

Very Very Low (rare but proven at least once)

- Blood Transfusion: 0.00004% estimated risk transmission from hospital blood transfusion
- Deep French kissing with oral sores (never well proven)
- Sharing sex toys (one report)

Zero

- Exposure to saliva, tears, hugs, shaking hands, shared personal objects, food or water
- Surface kissing
- HIV positive person on continuous, fully effective anti-HIV medication

CHAPTER 6
No Condom Sex with an HIV-Positive Person: Crazy?

In terms of HIV risk, what's safer for a woman?

A. Having sex — *without a condom* — with a HIV-positive man
   (the couple treated by an HIV knowledgeable doctor)?
B. Having a one-night stand — using condoms — with a random guy from a
   local nightclub?

ANSWER: A!
Here's why. Option A:
1. In this example, the man has HIV, the woman does not have HIV — the
   expected transmission of HIV per episode of vaginal intercourse is 8/10,000.
2. The HIV knowledgeable doctor in the above example makes sure the male is
   fully treated with ART, and the woman is protected with PrEP.
3. The chance an otherwise healthy HIV-positive male on effective ART passes
   HIV via unprotected vaginal intercourse approaches zero. For the sake of this
   discussion, let's take the *statistical worst scenario*, that transmission risk is
   lowered by 99.9 percent.
4. The woman would get a PrEP prescription, especially if there was even a
   sliver of doubt about the male's commitment to taking the ART as directed
   and staying current with all viral-load testing. If she is religious about taking
   her daily preventative mini-cocktail, her already negligible risk of contracting
   HIV goes down by another 99-plus percent.

So, the 8/10,000 chance an untreated HIV-positive male passing the virus during
one-night stand of unprotected vaginal intercourse is 99.9 percent reduced by
ART and in addition, 99-plus percent reduced by PrEP.

This worse case calculates out to less than a *one in hundred million chance* of
contracting HIV — one tenth the chance of dying from a lightning bolt this year.

Option B:
1. Of the 1.1 million HIV-positive Americans, 850,000 are men. About half are heterosexual or bisexual. About two-thirds are unaware of their diagnosis or untreated or inadequately treated.
2. For the sake of this discussion, let's assume there are 250,000 single inadequately treated HIV-positive heterosexual or bisexual men.
3. Assume there are 50,000,000 males in the heterosexual "dating" world, and that 250,000 are potentially at risk to spread HIV heterosexually, either because they are unaware of their diagnosis or inadequately treated but mistakenly convinced HIV cannot be transferred if condoms are used.
4. Condoms are not fail-safe. Estimates of screw-ups range from 5 percent to 40 percent. The failure rate with pregnancy prevention is 20 percent. The same is presumed for HIV protection.
5. Other common STDs — HSV, chlamydia and trichomonas — increase HIV transmission three-to-four-fold, and the majority of persons with these STDs are unaware of their infections.

So, there is about a 1 in 200 chance (250,000 divided by 50,000,000) that a random male partner will be HIV positive and either inadequately treated or unaware of his disease.

A 20 percent chance the condom won't "work."

A little less than 8 in 10 thousand chance an untreated HIV-positive male passes the virus to a woman if the condom breaks or falls off.

This calculates out to a less than one-in-a-million chance of contracting HIV.

So, in terms of getting HIV, it's 100-times safer for a woman to have sex with *no condom* with an HIV-positive man (both under a knowledgeable doctor's care) than having a one-night stand *using condoms* with a random hookup!

**In terms of getting HIV, it's 100-times safer for a woman to
have sex with no condom with an HIV-positive man
(both under a knowledgeable doctor's care) than having a
one-night stand using condoms with a random hookup!**

Unfortunately, two-thirds of those with HIV in the U.S. — approximately 750,000 individuals — are not treated or not treated optimally. As a result, there are 37,000 new infections and 6,700 deaths each year — all preventable.

Shockingly, in terms of numbers of deaths, HIV is not the worst STD.

That distinction goes to human papilloma virus (HPV).

CHAPTER 7
Human Papilloma Virus (HPV): The Quiet Killer

HPV has quietly become the most common — and the most deadly — STD in America. HIV caused 6,700 American fatalities in 2017; HPV killed twice that number.

HPV's rocket ride to "STD Killer" No.1 has been fueled by several very contagious strains which have the uncanny ability to infiltrate skin cell DNA and cause silent precancerous cell changes - which on occasion lead to invasive cancer.

HIV caused 6,700 American fatalities in 2017.

HPV killed twice that number.

The term epidemic hardly does the human papilloma virus justice. HPV is so common and so infectious that as many as 50 percent of college students test positive shortly after initiating sexual activity. During the first half year of a new relationship, couples typically transmit every strain they possess. Consequently, many persons with only one partner have HPV. Eventually, nine out of ten sexually active Americans will get this virus, then proceed to pass it on in ignorant bliss. Until 2006, the spread of HPV was unstoppable. Infectious disease experts were at their wits end. What do you tell high school teens in sex ed class when you know none of yesteryear's ABCs of STD control —abstinence, be faithful and condoms— work all that well?

Then in 2006, the breakthrough arrived – an extremely effective HPV vaccine. In 2012, an improved edition was released. End of story, right? No! Astonishingly, even among adolescents and young adults who would benefit most, far less than half have taken either vaccine. Americans remain eerily uninformed.

HPV is a close-knit family of 147 strains, all readily transmitted by skin to skin contact — with or without intercourse. All strains live exclusively in the epidermis (top layer of the skin). Based on unique DNA blueprints, each strain has its own favorite infection site and presentation. One hundred and ten HPV strains infect hand, foot and body skin — "regular" HPV. Thirty-seven are peeping-Tom "oro-genital" strains, existing only in delicate human scrotal, penile or outer vulvar skin or moist nasal, mouth, lung, inner eye lid, cervical, vaginal, anal or urethra linings.

Without the unwitting aid of host skin cell "machinery," HPV would not be able to make copies of itself and spread — much less survive. Immediately after gaining entry into epidermal cells, the virus sets up shop, hijacking human enzymes to make HPV proteins, including several known to handcuff DNA safety controls. This occasionally leads to unrestrained cell growth and sinister precancerous cells. Almost always, our immune system detects and eliminates these HPV-altered cells. About 10 percent of the time though, infected cells are not identified and destroyed, resulting in a persistent HPV infection.

Oro-genital HPV strains fall into two broad categories:

1. *Low-risk nuisance strains* (19 out of 37 known genital HPV strains) can cause warts but rarely if ever induce cancer. Types 6 and 11 cause 90 percent of anal, genital and bronchial airway warts.
2. *High-risk scary strains* (18 out of 37 known genital HPV strains) can cause microscopic intracellular "pre-cancer" cellular changes — initially invisible to the eye — which in a decade or two can morph into invasive knocking-on-heaven's-door cancer. Types 16 and 18 are responsible for 70 percent of HPV cancers.

How many Americans catch a new oro-genital HPV strain(s) each year?

14,000,000 (half are high-risk strains).

350,000 Americans get obvious oro-genital warts each year (all are low-risk strains).

How many Americans currently have oro-genital HPV?

79 million currently have one or more HPV strains at one or multiple sites on the body.

90 plus percent of Americans will get one or multiple HPV strains by age 50.

"Everybody has HPV, OK? Everybody has it. It's OK. Come out already. Everybody has it. If you don't have it yet, you go and get it. It's coming.

You don't have HPV yet? You're a fucking loser then, all right?"

— Ali Wong, 2016 / Baby Cobra, Netflix Comedy Special

11,000,000 American men (12 percent) and 3,000,000 American women (3 percent) have one or more oral HPV strains. Men who have sex with men (MSM) are exceptionally susceptible to oral HPV — 22 percent have current infections with high-risk strains.

How is HPV spread?

You catch HPV during skin-to-skin contact. HPV penetrates mucous membranes most readily but can also pass directly through intact skin. This minute virus — too small to even be seen by a regular microscope — readily jumps from infected to uninfected skin. During a single episode of vaginal sex, the chance of transmission is about 1 in 200 (so it's five-fold more infectious than HIV). Many persons are infected with multiple HPV strains, so their chance per sex act of spreading HPV is greater than 1 in 200. Understandably, HPV transmission is facilitated if the skin is abraded from pubic hair removal or from friction associated with sex.

Condoms, if faithfully and correctly used, limit HPV's access to most of the penis, but that still leaves a lot of open territory — genital, lower abdominal, inner thigh and anal regions. Not surprisingly, studies show condoms can only prevent about 50 percent of HPV transmissions.

Condoms limit HPV's access to most of the penis, but that still leaves a lot of open territory!

Condoms can only prevent about 50 percent of HPV transmissions.

Fingertips and sex toys can silently harbor infectious HPV. You can also occasionally get HPV from supposedly "safe" romantic encounters like petting, stroking, fingering and mutual masturbation. You can even possibly "auto-inoculate" HPV during masturbation from your own fingers to your own genitals. The virus is not spread through blood or body fluids.

Warts: The First Visible Evidence of Oro-Genital HPV

In the first weeks after contact, every HPV infection is invisible and symptomless. Early warning signs — cell changes caused by active viral replication — can only be seen in a microscope.

Months later, 5 percent of low-risk "nuisance" HPV infections sprout visible warts – much to the dismay of over 350,000 Americans each year. Genital warts have completely different looks depending on the strain and the outbreak location. On genital skin, HPV warts vary from dry crusty, to hard-to-spot tiny brown dots, to flat mole-like pigmented growths, to cauliflower topped lesions.

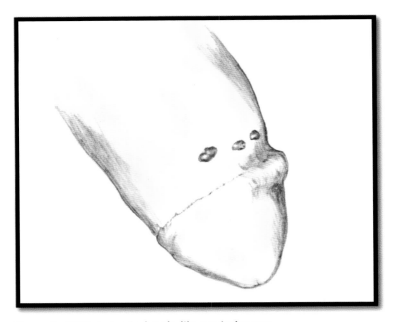

Figure 3 - HPV pigmented mole-like genital warts

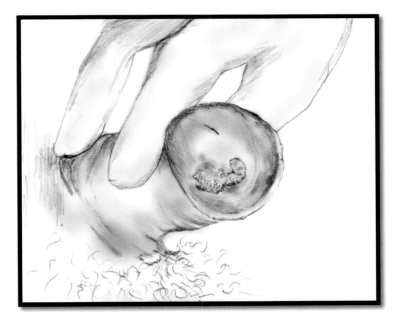

Figure 4 - Large HPV genital wart with cauliflower-top appearance

Mucous membrane warts in and around the vagina, urethra or anus are pale, boggy dots or slightly larger reddish cauliflower topped lesions or occasionally innocuous flat whitish plaques.

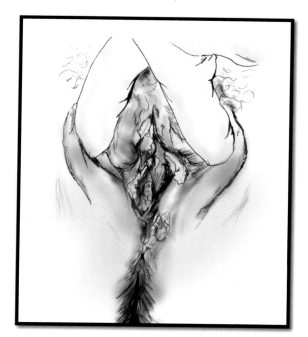

Figure 5 - HPV cauliflower topped warts in and around the vagina

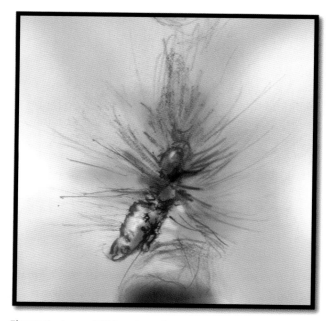

Figure 6 - Large HPV peri-anal warts

Genital warts also occasionally present inside the nose and inside the mouth.

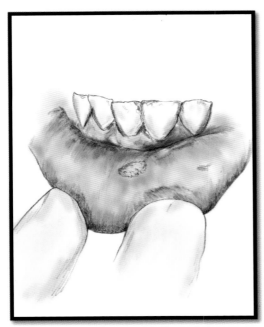

Figure 7- HPV oral wart with flat pale base

Foot HPV — plantar warts — known to persist on bathroom floors for days, are "non-genital" HPV warts (even though they occasionally infect bare footed lovers sharing a shower) and out of the scope of this discussion.

From a patient's perspective, each wart variety is equally ugly. All patients want them instantly gone — even if it takes sandblasting. Back in the '90s, I willingly acquiesced, relying on liquid nitrogen freezing, chemical burning or electric cautery to annihilate every last accessible penile, scrotal, abdominal, vulvar or perianal wart. For good measure, I'd cover the skin with vinegar-soaked 4x4 gauze pads – a trick to make even miniscule warts swell. These zapping treatments hurt, but that pain pales in comparison to the agony some women with multiple "out of sight" vaginal, cervical and urethral warts had to endure. They got tortured – literally. The 1990s gynecologic standard of care for procedure-happy doctors? A "scorched earth" chemical burn or laser of the entire vaginal cavity. OUCH!

Problem was, despite the full-court press, HPV invariably survived! The arrival of sensitive HPV DNA probes proved that even when all visible lesions were eradicated, the treated skin still intermittently shed replicating HPV! "Treated" patients remained infectious!

I was forced to rethink my anti-wart stance. Wart-burning therapies have cosmetic benefit, but HPV is not eliminated and patients are not healthier and probably are not less infectious. Warts are asymptomatic. Most warts resolve spontaneously in a year or two. Most importantly, warts are not harbingers of cancer. Why treat warts — and the patients they are attached to — so brutally?

Warts are not harbingers of cancer. Why treat warts – and the patients they are attached to – so brutally?

Wary of over the top treatments, I now tell patients: *"warts are no big deal."* I still recommend exterminating cosmetically egregious lesions but that's it. Symptoms that do crop up — itching, pain, vaginal discharge or bleeding — are invariably not signs of warts. They could however, be red flags for other STDs. Burning with urination is often another red flag symptom, but rarely, it is in fact due to HPV. Five percent of warts present in the urethra (17,500 cases per year), and many of these set up shop at the tip of the urethra and may cause stinging during urination.

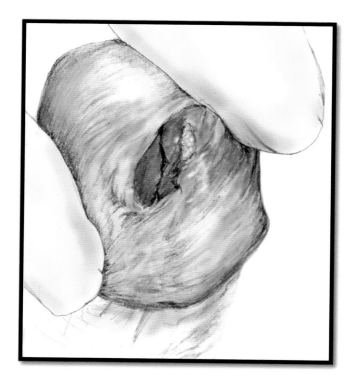

Figure 8 - Top of the penis with the urethral tip retracted open to reveal HPV wart

HPV can spread up the urethra all the way to the bladder or, rarely, Foley catheter insertion "seeds" the virus up the urethra. (I've seen this complication once. It was not pretty.) Its best to treat these warts, but no one knows if burning the visible urethral lesions will in fact prevent future "seeding" from adjacent invisible HPV infections.

Similar seeding issues need to be considered before sigmoidoscopes and colonoscopes are inserted up the rectum potentially spreading existing peri- and intra-anal warts. Immuno-suppressed persons — transplant patients, cancer chemo patients, those with HIV infection or diabetics — in addition to being more likely to get persistent HPV infections, tend to get multiple strains of warts that spread around the anus, even with no prior rectal intercourse. Intra-anal warts, on the other hand, are only seen in MSM or heterosexual women who practice receptive anal intercourse.

What is the most ruthless HPV wart?

Hands down, the most ruthless wart is respiratory papillomatosis. It's transmitted during vaginal delivery to about 500 American newborns each year. HPV acquired during childbirth can result in multiple warty growths inside the delicate baby bronchial tubes. These typically stay unnoticed until respiratory problems, fatal in rare instances, emerge as the warts sometimes grow to a critical size around age 2, partially obstructing breathing tubes.

Genital Warts	HPV Strains
Respiratory papillomatosis "the most ruthless wart"	6, 11
Eye conjunctival papillomas	6, 11
Sinus papilloma	57
Genital warts	6, 11

Table 5

How does HPV turn into cancer?

Within a year of first having sex, up to 40 percent of Americans are infected with a cancer-causing HPV strain (i.e. especially strains 16, 18, and 45). These strains are tagged "high-risk" based on their ability to silently infiltrate into skin cell DNA, inactivate genes which safeguard orderly cell growth and potentially transform skin cells over many years into cancer. For instance, cervical cancer cells contain strain 16 about 50 percent of the time ("high-risk") whereas HPV strain 4 is identified in cervical cancer cells about 0.1 percent of the time ("low-risk"). Wart-inducing HPV strains almost never cause cancer, hence their low-risk, cosmetic-only label.

Within the first year or two of every high-risk HPV infection, subtle pre-cancer changes are seen if the affected tissue is examined under a microscope. Early cervix surface changes are documented as low-level PAP smear abnormalities. Similar pathologic changes occur in infected vulvar, anal and posterior tongue/tonsillar tissue.

Finally, the body's immune system at long last steps in, specific anti-HPV antibodies are formed, and within two years, 90 percent of the time the offending strain is eliminated or at least deep-sixed into hibernation (non-replicating "latent" infection if you want the exact medical lingo). Either way, HPV DNA can no longer be detected on the skin surface. Simultaneously, the corresponding pre-cancerous tissue changes disappear. For reasons that still have experts flummoxed, about 10 percent of the time, the body's immune system fails to eradicate HPV, allowing HPV carte blanche to replicate unperturbed, and as time elapses, induce pre-cancer cell changes closer and closer to cancer.

Cancers (U.S.)	% of Cancer Caused by HPV	Cancer Incidence/yr.	Deaths/yr.
Cervical	95	13,788	4,210
Oropharyngeal	Female 70	3,438	576
	Male 70	15,479	2,377
Vulvar	70	6,020	1,150
Vaginal	85	4,810	1,240
Penile	65	2,120	360
Anal	Female 95	3,200	576
	Male 95	2,950	450
Mouth	Unknown		
Esophageal	Unknown		
Genital Skin (Bowen's Disease)	Unknown		
Bladder	Unknown		
Lung	Unknown		
Total U.S.		50,000	11,000
Cervical Cancer Worldwide, (2012)		445,000	270,000

(85% of cervical cancer deaths occur in low and middle-income countries)

Table 6

Each year, more than 50,000 Americans get full blown HPV cancer. One in five will die. In the midst of this deadly HPV rampage, the PAP smear — a clever test formulated in the 1920s by Greek pathologist, Dr. George Papanicolaou — has been a veritable life savior. He microscopically examined cervix cell scrapings obtained during pelvic exams and discovered that the type and extent of cervical cell abnormality telegraphs the degree of cancer risk.

In increasing order of severity, these are the possible results of your PAP:

1.   Normal

2.   Atypical squamous cells of unknown significance (ASCUS)

3.   Low-Grade Squamous Intraepithelial Lesion (LGSIL)

4.   High-Grade Squamous Intraepithelial Lesion (HGSIL).

If the PAP goes from normal one year to HGSIL the next year, this severe abnormality needs to be surgically removed. If left untreated, 35 percent of woman will develop invasive cervical cancer over the ensuing 10 - 20 years (rarely, HGSIL progresses to cancer in as little as 3 years).

5.   Cervical Cancer

If no PAP smear is ever done, the life time risk of cervical cancer is about 2 percent – the risk doubles to 4 percent if a woman has ever been positive for a high-risk HPV strain.

Hands down, the PAP smear has been the most effective cancer-screening test of all time. Even less than optimal use of PAP tests over the last 30 years has dropped the risk of dying from cervical cancer by ten-fold, saving tens of thousands of women's lives each year. If used properly across the world, the PAP smear has the potential to save hundreds of thousands of women's lives.

But the lifesaving annual PAP smear - based on eye opening results from a 2018 Canadian study - may soon be a relic of our past! Amazingly, screening the cervix for high risk HPV strains is more effective than regular PAP's in preventing cervical cancer, even when performed only once every 5 years.

Currently, experts recommend one of the following three cervical cancer prevention approaches:
   a) High risk HPV testing of the cervix every 5 years
      This is the best cervical cancer detection method; the downside is that initially this approach has more false positive results so more testing (colposcopies) needs to be done compared to the PAP smear only approach.

b) Cervical PAP smear every 3 years

This approach is predicted to to result in slightly more cervical cancer deaths than the every 5 year HPV screening 8 vs. 3 deaths per 10,000 women. Women who don't do any screening can expect a 10 to 30-fold higher chance of dying from cervical cancer.

c) Co-testing - PAP smear plus high risk HPV testing every 5 years

This a less effective strategy than the above two choices based on increased cost and procedures.

All women aged 21 to 29 should continue to do PAP smears every 3 years then begin one of the above protocols at age 30 (HPV testing can be initiated at age 25 for women who begin sex before before age 18). Screening is not recommended for women younger than 21 or low risk women older than 65 with multiple prior negative cervical screenings. It also isn't recommended for those who've had their cervix surgically removal. For now, women who have received HPV vaccination should follow the above protocols despite being at much lower risk of precancerous changes.

Interpreting either "positive" or "negative" results for high-risk strains can be confusing.

Negative HPV means you currently have no detectable replicating (active) DNA from any of the 14 tested cancer-causing strains. Either you've never been infected or you were infected in the past but you are one of the fortunate individuals where the high-risk HPV strain has spontaneously cleared.
Positive HPV in the new *cobas®* *HPV test* means you currently have one or more active infection(s) from either:

a) strain 16

b) strain 18

c) one of the other 12 high-risk strains detected in the cobas® test.

Positive high-risk HPV is a warning, not a signal of imminent danger or cancer. Remember, 90 percent of these infections spontaneously clear in a year or two. On the other hand, a word of caution. The PAP smear is not perfect. One in ten women with normal PAP smears — and a positive HPV 16 or 18 test — in fact really have deleterious cervical cell changes that their initial PAP smear missed.

Doctors cannot treat positive HPV results – there is currently no anti-viral drug to eradicate HPV. Doctors can treat associated warts, abnormal cell changes or overt cancers. So, the effect of a positive high-risk HPV result on top of a normal PAP is to do more frequent repeat screens or more aggressive exams (i.e. colposcopy). Always be cognizant of possible sampling errors. PAP changes may not reflect the "most advanced" changes. If mild PAP changes are seen with a persistently positive high-risk strain, there is a rationale to look more extensively for cancer. If the PAP is normal, repeat testing in 6 - 12 months for the high-risk strain usually makes the most sense. Often, the high-risk strain will spontaneously disappear.

DOCTORS H AND K RECOMMEND:

Understand the difference between the high-risk HPV test of the cervix and the PAP smear, a test to look for cellular changes of the cervix.

Beginning in women 30 years of age, HPV testing is often appropriate every 5 years instead of the PAP smear. Make sure you ask your doctor if you are getting the HPV DNA test (the best screening test) or the HPV messenger RNA test (an inferior screening test no longer recommended).

Cunnilingus Cancer

Michael Douglas put HPV throat cancer on the map in a historic 2013 *Guardian* newspaper interview. Asked whether he now regretted his years of smoking and drinking — formerly thought to be the cause of all oral cancers — Michael Douglas stunned the world with his shockingly honest reply:

> *"No. Because without wanting to get too specific, this particular cancer is caused by HPV, which actually comes about from cunnilingus."*

Just several decades ago, throat cancer (oral squamous cell carcinoma) was uncommon. When it appeared, booze and tobacco were to blame. Now everything's changed. Oral cancer is not rare: 18,917 cases (15,479 men; 3,438 women) occurred in America this year. In the wake of the HPV epidemic, oral cancer is increasing over the last 20 years at an unprecedented 3 percent yearly clip. Men are disproportionally affected. Individual strains known to contribute to head and neck cancer are six-fold higher in men (2 percent) than woman (0.3 percent). Cervical cancer is no longer America's most common HPV cancer; Oral cancer now takes that dubious distinction.

The salacious Michael Douglas claim — that he got oral HPV via cunnilingus with his ex-wife, then years later that virus triggered his oral cancer?

Possible? Yes.
Provable? No.

Here's why. First, it's likely there were other cunninglingus partners along the way years before Douglas's HPV-related oral cancer diagnosis in 2010. HPV-induced oral cancer takes at least 10 - 20 years after an initial HPV infection that doesn't spontaneously "clear." Second, assume his ex-wife indeed was "positive" for HPV. The fact is, there are 18 high-risk strains. Who says his and her strains match? Who says he didn't contract that particular viral strain elsewhere?

As it turned out, the ex-wife went public and declared her lady junk was HPV-free. OK, let's assume she did have a thorough medical exam and was told she was HPV free. A top notch private doctor's office lab can check for just 14 of the 18 high-risk HPV strains (some gynecology offices can just test for three high-risk strains). Let's go one step further. Even if she did go to a research center and tests showed she had NONE of the 18 known high-risk strains — that proves nothing. It does not mean she did not in the distant past have an infection with a high-risk strain. A *negative DNA HPV test today does not mean there was no past HPV infection!* Remember, the body clears 90 percent of HPV and 10 percent persists for longer than 2 years. A strain the ex-wife was able to quickly clear, may regrettably be transmitted and persist — later leading to oral cancer in her ex-husband — born with a less resourceful, less effective immune system.

Risk factors for HPV oral cancer:
1. Oral sex
2. Males: 400 percent increased risk compared to females
3. MSM: 300 percent increased risk compared to heterosexual men
4. Greater than 16 heterosexual partners: 20 percent greater risk
5. Cigarette use: 10 percent greater risk
6. Marijuana use: 6 percent greater risk
7. Heavy alcohol use
8. Impaired immune system (diabetes, poor oral hygiene, chronic inflammation and infections, diseases or drugs that suppress the body's immune system)

Male and female HPV rates are similar in genital regions – so why do men have a four-fold greater risk of HPV and HPV throat cancer compared to women?

The most likely explanation is that cunnilingus is four-fold riskier than fellacio in terms of acquiring high-risk HPV strains. Vaginal-to-mouth contact appears fellatio to be more infectious than penile-to-mouth fellatio because of increased mucous membrane to mucous membrane exposure in cunnilingus.

No one knows the infectivity of HPV via deep French kissing. However, if kissing was a major cause of oral HPV, you'd expect the male to female ratio to be much more equal.

How does throat cancer present?

Throat and tongue cancer creeps up like a stealth bomber. First, one of the high-risk strains is silently acquired via oral sex. Then a decade or two later, out of the blue, hoarseness, difficulty swallowing, non-healing lesions on the tongue, tonsil or top of the mouth, unexplained neck lumps or weight loss presents. Then — boom! — an explosive malignancy. Oral cancer and its treatment — surgery, chemotherapy and radiation therapy — are hellish: dry mouth, dental disease, inability to swallow, feeding tubes for nutrition, unintended weight loss. Just seeing one patient live through this nightmare heightens the urgency to prevent, or at least detect, oral cancer in its earliest stage.

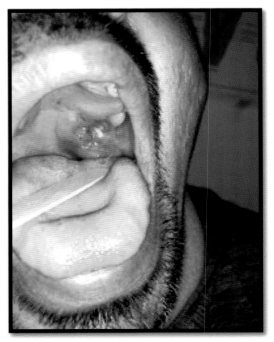

Figure 9 - HPV induced oral squamous cell cancer on the left tonsil
Photo courtesy of Dr. Uttam Sinha, MD, FACS

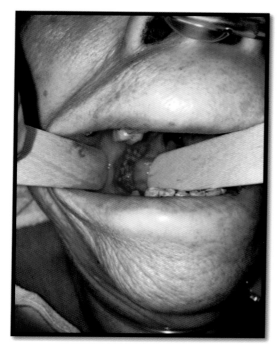

Figure 10 - HPV induced oral squamous cell cancer
Photo courtesy of Dr. Uttam Sinha, MD, FACS

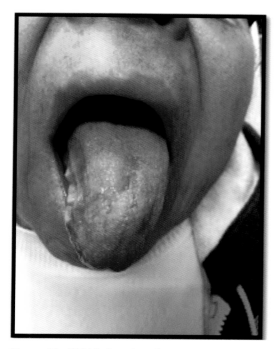

Figure 11 - HPV induced oral squamous cell cancer in the mid lateral tongue
Photo courtesy of Dr. Uttam Sinha, MD, FACS

Bottom line: Just like regular PAP smears in the past - and now every 5 year HPV testing - are critical for cervical cancer prevention, you've got to know the early signs of oral cancer. It can be treated better if caught early. The silver lining? HPV induced oral cancer responds to treatment better than "cigarette and booze" induced oral cancer.

Don't be a head-in-sand ostrich. If you get a sore throat, hoarseness or painless neck lump for no apparent reason for over a week – don't blow it off. Dude, it could be cunnilingus cancer!

Other Sexually Transmitted HPV Associated Cancers

Anal and rectal HPV related cancers are also rapidly increasing over the last 20 years. Especially hard hit are Americans in the 50 to 70 age group - anal and rectal cancer in this demographic is increasing over the last 2 decades at a shocking 5 percent per year! Anal cancer symptoms include an unexplained anal lump, pain or anal bleeding. MSM and heterosexual women who have receptive anal intercourse need a yearly anal finger exam.

Also worrisome, but not well studied, is the probable contribution of high risk genital HPV strains to squamous cell carcinomas of the lung (four-fold more common than cervical squamous cell carcinomas), esophagus and bladder.

Lastly, HPV occasionally causes slow growing red, brown or skin colored scaly patches on the lip, mouth or genital skin called "Bowen's Disease". These are associated with high risk HPV strains 16, 16, 34 and 48 and have a 5% chance of morphing to squamous skin cancer (Figure 12).

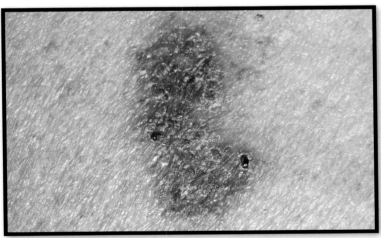

Figure 12 - This unusual scaly genital or lip lesion can easily be confused with eczema or psoriasis

Photo credit, NHS (UK) website

How is HPV Diagnosed?

Visual Diagnosis: People think you just need to look at the genitals to diagnose HPV. If you see warts, you've got HPV. Conversely, no warts — no HPV.

Geez! Single life would be so much easier if HPV was that straightforward!

In real life, most low risk strains remain invisible to the human eye. Only about 5 percent of new low-risk HPV infections present as easily seen warts. Additional warts masquerade as "normal' moles while others are hidden inside the anus, vagina, urethra or nasopharynx. Warts signal innocuous though unsightly and infectious HPV strains.

Unfortunately, high-risk strains initially have no tell-tale signs - the early cell changes are invisible to the human eye. You cannot diagnose cancer causing HPV strains visually... until it's way way too late!

Culture Diagnosis: Viral cultures are rarely if ever used - HPV is too difficult to grow in a test tube for there to be any practical value to this test.

Blood Tests: *HPV Antibody levels:* To successfully fight off HPV, your immune system has to recognize and then destroy literally tens of thousands of these foreign skin invaders. One way to accomplish this task is by white blood cells producing strain specific anti-HPV antibodies. Most people who "clear" HPV have high levels of these specific antibodies. Patients with persistent HPV infections have subpar immune systems unable to generate detectable anti-viral antibody.

Tissue Diagnosis:

a. Examine skin cells for HPV infection:
Rubbing a Q-tip over skin collects superficial cells just ready to be sloughed off. When the insides of these skin cells are "interrogated" by HPV DNA probes (unique pieces of genetic material attached to a column), it's possible to identify all skin locations infected with active, replicating HPV. This test can be done in research facilities for each of the 37 oral-genital HPV strains on any skin surface.

Gynecologists routinely use this approach to test cervical "skin" cells for HPV types 16, 18 and 45 – the high risk strains that cause 70-80 percent of HPV-associated cervical cancer. Recently, the cobas HPV test allows screening for 14 out of the 18 known high risk strains, accounting for over 90 percent of HPV-associated cervical cancer.

b. Examine skin cells microscopically for warts or HPV induced precancer or cancer:
Cells are obtained by:

a. PAP smear: Gently scrape off cervix surface cells and examine microscopically

b. Anal PAP: Gently scrape off anal surface cells and examine microscopically.

c. Biopsy: Surgically remove suspicious skin or mucous membrane lesions and examine microscopically

There are no viable screening methods similar to a cervical PAP test for detecting "Michael Douglas" throat cancer, but as you might imagine, it's an area of intense research. The cervix and back of tongue surface have a critical difference: The cervix surface is flat while the throat surface is uneven with crevasses and ridges. Consequently, cervical scrapings yield representative samples of surface cells. In the throat, scrapings produce mainly cells from the upper ridges. Unfortunately, throat cancer typically begins in the inaccessible "crevasses."

The surprising recent evidence showing that screening for HPV every 5 years is a more effective cervical cancer test than the yearly PAP raises hope that other cancers can also now be prevented with new state-of-the-art HPV probes. Specifically, should we now attack deadly anal, rectal, vulvar, oropharyngeal and esophageal cancer by sampling those surfaces for high risk HPV every 5 years? Should we just concentrate on high risk individuals? The hesitancy (an appropriate one in our opinion) is due to the fact these not yet approved anal and oral HPV tests have not yet been well tested as to their ability to prevent future cancer. My prediction is that HPV screening will be the standard of care for each of these cancers in the near future.

TAKE HOME LESSON FROM DOCTORS H AND K:

Be smart. Be careful. Non-FDA approved tests means that no regulatory agency has reviewed the test performance, its accuracy or its ability to detect or prevent disease.

Additionally, getting a non-FDA approved test (or drug) means your insurance company will not pay!

Sometimes the fact there is no approved HPV test for men makes it seem that HPV is a women disease. Nothing could be further from the truth.

Sometimes the fact there is no approved HPV test for men makes it seem that HPV is a women disease. Nothing could be further from the truth.

Is HPV Curable?

Partially. The body fights off and may "cure" or inactivate 90 percent of infections by producing antibodies that attack and kill this virus. However, no anti-viral drug or treatment is available if the body's immune system stumbles and fails to fully clear HPV.

Is HPV Treatable?

Yes.

Measures to boost the body's immune system — i.e. lose excess fat to treat diabetes, stop medication like steroids or take antibiotics or anti-virals to eliminate chronic infections like TB, Hepatitis or HIV — can assist HPV eradication.

Conversely, the effects of HPV infection are treatable. Visible genital warts can be eliminated by topical chemicals, excisional surgery, liquid nitrogen freezing or laser surgery. Once identified, abnormal cells or precancer on the cervix can be eliminated by cryosurgery (freezing), LEEP (loop electrosurgical excision procedure), conization (surgery with a scalpel to remove a cone-shaped piece of the cervical canal) and laser vaporization conization. Cancer can be surgically removed or if it has metastasized, treated with radiation and or chemotherapy.

What are my chances of catching HPV cancer?

The lifetime chance of each of us getting any invasive cancer is approximately 40 percent. HPV causes about 2 to 3 percent of these cancers. So, your lifetime risk of getting an HPV induced invasive cancer is 1 percent. This number could go much higher if in the future HPV was shown to be responsible for some portion of squamous cell carcinoma of the lungs, esophagus or bladder.

Women with a one-time documented high-risk HPV strain infection have a 3 - 4 percent lifetime risk of cervical cancer. Women with persistent high-risk strain(s) have a 30 percent lifetime risk of invasive cervical cancer. Long-term birth control pill use and having multiple children further increase cervical cancer risk.

Is HPV Preventable?

Yes, yes, yes!

Awareness is prevention

To combat HPV, understand that this virus doesn't play fair. It silently and deliberately induces nearly 50,000 new cancers each year in the USA alone. By the time symptoms appear — a neck bump first felt while shaving, an itchy vulvar lump or post-intercourse vaginal bleeding — the cancer can be widely metastatic.

Doctors H and K have seen many HPV cancers in their careers.

The gut-wrencher? These killer cancers are more than 90 percent preventable.

Parents: Understand the medical gravity of infectious disease epidemics your children face and respond accordingly. For instance, many colleges mandate a meningococcal vaccine for incoming freshman. Given repeated deadly campus outbreaks, this policy is defensible. But these vaccines at best can prevent 200 deaths per year.

With HPV, we're talking about *hundreds of thousands* of preventable genital warts. We're talking about *hundreds of thousands* of cervical procedures mandated by an abnormal PAP, which causes untold anxiety and expense; complications can even occasionally affect fertility. And we're talking about *tens of thousands* of invasive cancers, toxic cancer treatments and potential deaths.

If parents recognize these grim statistics, I doubt they'll continue to leave the majority of their children unvaccinated – and unprotected.

Prophylaxis is prevention: The HPV Vaccine

In 2006, a highly effective HPV vaccine, Gardasil® 4, protecting against wart (6, 11) and cancer (16, 18) strains was approved. Hallelujah!

This is an amazing accomplishment. In stark contrast, a herpes vaccine was touted as being "just around the corner" 50 years ago – and still has not materialized. Other vaccines, most notably HIV, remain just as elusive.

The current 2012 edition, Gardasil® 9, is constructed from single proteins from HPV 6, 11 — accounting for 90 percent of genital warts — and 16, 18, 31, 33, 45, 52 and 58 — accounting for over 75 to 85 percent of cervical cancer. The secret sauce is strain-specific proteins mixed with an aluminum adjuvant that elicits the production of protective antibodies in more than 99 percent of persons.

The HPV vaccine is optimally given in a series of two shots to boys and girls around the age of 12 or a series of three shots for young adults age 15 to 26, *even if they've already had sex*. Though HPV infection typically happens soon after intimacy begins, a person might not be exposed to all of the 9 HPV types that are in the vaccine. Early vaccinations allow time to build an immune response in advance of HPV exposure and produce a higher immune response in preteens compared with older teens and adults. Ten years after the vaccine, there's been no evidence of waning protection, so as of now, no booster shots are needed.

The single viral proteins in the vaccine can never initiate an infection. Likewise, the vaccine has no effect against established HPV infections.

Studies clearly show preteens and teens who receive this vaccine do not have sex any sooner or any more frequently than unvaccinated classmates. The HPV vaccine is not a trapdoor to promiscuity.

Studies in Australia show that after six years, vaccinated subjects not only have "protective" antibodies, but those antibodies actually prevent each type of HPV included in the vaccine. There was no increase in non-vaccinated strains. Most importantly, the vaccine at six years lived up to its hype! A huge drop in genital warts and cervical precancers was documented. It takes at least 10 years for HPV cancer to develop, so confirmation of expected reductions of new cervical, vulvar, anal and oral cancer will have to wait a number of years.

Hepatitis B Vaccine Reveals the Enormous Potential of HPV Vaccine

Worldwide, 1.4 million cancers are caused by viral infections. The lion's share of those cancers is caused by Human papilloma virus (600,000 cases) and Hepatitis B virus (380,000 cases).

Studies over the last 25 years on the effects of the Hep B vaccine reveal the stunning potential of the HPV vaccine.

Hepatis B virus — spread via sex, blood exposure and childbirth like HIV, but ten-fold more contagious — currently infects about 240 million people worldwide. 25 to 40 percent of these cases will go on to develop fatal cirrhosis or liver cancer if treatment is not available, potentially resulting in 786,000 deaths each year.

In the last several decades, more than 1 billion doses of Hepatitis B vaccine have been administered worldwide — mostly to infants. In Taiwan, a country where more than 15 percent of children got hepatitis B, universal vaccination

---

programs begun 25 years ago have lowered that number by 95 percent and more importantly, lowered the number of Hep B associated liver cancers in young adults by a similar percent.

Crunching the numbers, based on the intensive worldwide Hepatitis B vaccine push from 2000 - 2011, an estimated *3.7 million deaths have been prevented.* Yes! Hepatitis B is the world's first successful "cancer vaccine"!

Preliminary evidence indicates that the HPV vaccine will be the second successful cancer vaccine with the potential to even exceed the Hep B vaccine's spectacular lifesaving ability.

Under optimal circumstances, the HPV vaccine could avert hundreds of thousands of deaths while saving the health care system untold billions by preventing most of the following medical conditions:
- HPV genital warts (350,000 U.S. cases per year)
- HPV cancer (40,000-50,000 U.S. cases per year)
- Cervical pre-cancers (300,000 U.S. cases per year endure invasive testing and prophylactic treatment that occasionally causes preterm labor or delivery problems)
- Fatal infant throat and lung warts (500 plus babies per year)

Doctors H and K firmly believe:

Once parents understand what's at stake,
they will run, not walk,
their kids in for the HPV vaccine series.

HPV Vaccine Safety

The HPV vaccine is relatively expensive ($400), but it's covered by insurers. Given the stakes, even if you had to pay cash, it's a bargain-basement price. As with the Hep B vaccine, the costs for low and middle-income countries have dropped to less than 5 dollars per HPV shot, giving hope that in the not too distant future, the worldwide cervical cancer epidemic, killing hundreds of thousands of women, will end.

There is no side-effect-free drug or surgical procedure — or vaccine. Brief injection site reactions to Gardasil® 4 or Gardasil® 9 are not uncommon. The injection site hurts and there is occasionally 24 - 48 hours of mild fever,

venturing out into the singles market. She's doesn't qualify for the vaccine? Are you kidding me?

Clinical trial data shows that the HPV vaccine is safe and immunogenic in women (and presumably men) at least up to the age of 55. HPV vaccination in individuals over 26 is officially recommended in several countries. HPV vaccination is likely to be beneficial to sexually active older men and women due to their continuous risk of acquiring new HPV infections and of developing oral, cervical or other types of HPV induced cancer. Obviously, vaccination benefits shrink with advancing age – more past partners, more ongoing HPV infections and weaker immune systems.

OK, I'm not that stupid. I realize the HPV vaccine efficacy and safety were only scientifically studied in persons under 26, therefore, the vaccine advisory committee's sage "guidelines." That being said, here are my practical recommendations:

1. Individuals older than 26 should be offered vaccination when contemplating a new sexual relationship on a case by case basis.

2. Give Gardasil® 9 vaccine to those at especially high-risk of HPV disease if less than 55 and beginning a new relationship.
   a. gay and bisexual men (MSM)
   b. individuals with weakened immune systems, i.e. diabetics, autoimmune disease, transplant or cancer patients and those with chronic infections like TB and HIV

Real Cases: Real Confusion, Real Questions

This 23-year-old patient of mine and her best friend personify real world out-of-control HPV confusion.

She arrives in my office, a copy of her recent *normal* PAP test in hand. But she also shows me her "co-test" results – positive for HPV 18 despite claiming to have had the full Gardasil® 4 series! Her gynecologist just told her HPV 18 is a cervical cancer-causing strain that persists for a lifetime and pushed her to immediately do a colposcopy: a special examination using magnifying scope to examine the cervix and biopsy any pre-cancer surface changes.

She freaked and ran for a second opinion.

Beverly Hills gynecologist #2 told her, "HPV is transient. It should disappear in a year or two. No big deal. Repeat the PAP in a year. In fact, the HPV test should never have been done in the first place; it's only for women over 30 years old!"

A possible cancer? Or nothing to worry about? Hearing two opposite opinions – from two swanky Beverly Hills doctors – freaks her out even more. She schedules an appointment with me on an urgent basis and pleads, *"Which recommendation should I take?"*

Me: "Gynecologist #2 is right... except that HPV is *almost always* transient. Ten percent of the time it persists. Gynecologist #2 correctly notes the consensus, HPV testing should not be initiated till age 30. Perhaps an exception where HPV screening might be considered at age 25 - an unvaccinated woman who began sex at an early age.

Bottom line: We treat the cervical cell changes – not the HPV infection! And a normal PAP means no cervical changes. After age 30, however, doctors get nervous if there is persistent high-risk HPV detected. So, they may then proceed directly to colposcopy even in the face of a normal PAP. This is because the PAP smear is "falsely" normal (looking at the entire cervix surface with colposcopy would find a pathological pre-cancer abnormality) up to 10 percent of the time. Whew. So yes, just relax! And do a follow-up co-test in 12 months

She had a slew of follow-up questions: *"Why do I have HPV 18 – I got the vaccine?!?"*

Given that the HPV vaccines are 99 percent effective against HPV strain 18, is she the unlucky 1 out of 100? Possibly, but consider most adolescents still cling to the Bill Clinton definition of sex. One likely explanation in this case was episodes of genital touching or oral sex before full vaccine administration. A second explanation is the strain was transient. It will go away when she is retested one year later. Remember the vaccine is best at protecting against persistent infection, not specifically initial infection.

How come my ex-boyfriend was routinely vaccinated as a child and my current guy's doctor told him the HPV vaccine was not indicated?

Your current guy is older, the CDC did not recommend males get HPV vaccines until 2011, and then they said not to give it to males over 21. Those recommendations don't seem correct to me but not all doctors administer vaccines on a case-by-case basis; some just follow the CDC's recommendations to a T. Actually, much of the issue is regarding insurance coverage. Until the CDC officially endorses a vaccines use, most insurers will not pay for it.

Is there any truth in those internet sites swearing the HPV vaccine has terrible possible side effects?

No. We cannot rule out a one-in-a-million chance but look at the worst-case scenario: a small number of people might get serious side effects while tens of thousands would have cancer prevented. The risk-to-reward ratio is exceedingly tilted to the reward side. I took the HPV vaccine myself after the age of 50.

My 23-year-old patient left that night for a planned vacation. The very next day, while naturally soaking up vitamin D on an isolated third world beach, her 24-year-old girlfriend hysterically calls. Her PAP just returned abnormal "LSIL pre-cancer" even though she had gotten the Gardasil® 4 after her first boyfriend. She was told to set up a colposcopy and possible cancer surgery ASAP! My 23-year-old patient urges her to confer immediately with her second opinion gynecologist and me. The second opinion doctor says, "Just take Gardasil® 9, repeat the PAP in one year and relax. The 'LSIL' changes almost always go away in someone 24-years-old."

Cancer surgery? Or just relax? Those are diametrically different opinions! She comes into my office on an emergency basis, literally sweating bullets. What should the friend do?

Again, I side with gynecologist #2. Relax!

Her LSIL changes are due to a cervical HPV infection from a high-risk strain - an extremely common finding at age 24 (about 20 percent). There is a 90 percent chance the abnormal PAP will resolve over the next one to two years. A co-test (a PAP and an HPV viral test) in one year is appropriate.

What about her vaccination history? Is she protected since she had taken Gardasil® 4?

I commonly hear some variation of this story... *"I got Gardasil® 4 vaccine before I had too many partners..."* Given high rates of transmission within six months of a relationship, you often get one or more HPV strains from your very first partner, especially if they were more "experienced."

"Should I get Gardasil® 9 even though I got Gardasil® 4?"

The younger you are, the fewer the number of past partners, the more common your use of condoms, the more emphatically I will answer this question yes.

I've had a lot of oral sex. If I have cervical pre-cancer, could I have oral pre-cancer too? Is there a test for that?

The first step: do you have special oral HPV induced throat cancer risk factors? Are you an MSM? A heterosexual man with greater that 16 lifetime partners? Do you smoke cigarettes or marijuana? Use excessive amounts of alcohol? Have an impaired immune system?

An oral gargle spit test is available but not FDA-approved. I use it occasionally but God forbid the test shows high risk HPV is present. Patients get extremely anxious when learning they have a cancer-causing virus but there's no known treatment. Scrapings of surface cells won't detect the early cancers. We can set up serial throat exams and or larygoscopies but we don't know whether this can effectively prevent cancer.

Literally that same week, I see a patient who has been told by a very respectable Beverly Hills dermatologist to get multiple penile and peri-anal warts (which don't bother him in any way) removed because:

   a) they are a risk to later turn cancerous

   b) they pose a risk to spread to his partner

No! Bad advice! I see the patient and very frankly, I am uncertain he even has warts! Not everything in medicine is black or white - in this case I told him there was a 50% chance he had tiny warts and a 50% chance he had benign tags - the only way to know for sure would be to do an HPV scraping or a biopsy and examine the skin under the microscope.

Bottom line, if in fact he even had genital HPV warts, removing them probably would not decrease his infectivity - too many other small or invisible lesions left behind. Genital warts are not cancerous so no need to remove on that basis. The only reason to proceed was if these warts were cosmetically objectionable. They were not. I told him to go home and stop pubic grooming! Abraded skin allows easy access inside the body to HPV - as well as other skin to skin STDs like syphilis and herpes.

Genital HPV Summary:
   1. Increased HPV transmission:
      a. Skin or mucous membrane abrasions, irritations, cuts or sores
         i. Post intercourse (friction area above the condom rim opposite the female's mons pubis is common fertile ground for HPV)
         ii. Shaving/hair removal (up to 400 percent increased transmission)
         iii. Other infections like genital herpes that affect integrity of mucous membranes
      b. Medical Procedures
         i. Tube up to bladder (cystoscopy) if urinary HPV
         ii. Tube up anus (colonoscopy) if perianal or anal HPV
         iii. Vaginal Delivery: If vaginal warts, a newborns first breaths rarely inhale shedding HPV, resulting in throat and lung warts (respiratory papillomatosis)

    c. Moisture (with weight gain in pubic regions where skin touching skin)

    d. Cigarettes (smoking also speeds progression of mild to more severe abnormal PAP smears)

    e. Multiple sex partners

    f. Newly acquired HPV infections more contagious

    g. Immunosuppression (diabetic, cancer, transplant or AIDS patients, or persons on immune suppressing meds)

2. Decreased HPV transmission:

    a. Abstinence (this is not foolproof: hand to genital touching can spread HPV)

    b. Vaccination (maximal effectiveness in individuals younger than 14 at height of vaccine responsiveness and before any sexual activity)

    c. Condoms (partial protection)

    d. Circumcision (partial protection)

3. Possibly spread by:

    a. Fomites - toilet seats, gym machines, floors - occasional sources for non-genital warts and rarely for genital warts

    b. Damp towels – documented case of transfer of HPV strain from sexually active girl to two virginal girls who lived together in dormitory and occasionally shared towels after showers

4. Not spread by:

    a. Blood

    b. Body fluids

    c. Swimming pools or hot tubs

    d. Sharing food or utensils

5. HPV associated cancer prevention

    a. Primary high risk HPV testing on cervical surface every 5 years beginning at age 30

    b. Pap smear (cervical cell scraping) every 3 years beginning age 21

    c. HPV testing on other tissues (anal, vulvar, penile, oral or esophageal) makes logical sense but is still of unproven value for cancer prevention

CHAPTER 8
Hairless Hygiene: Smooth on the Outside, Infected Inside?

When I began doctoring, everyone over twelve had pubic hair.

Today, in my Beverly Hills practice, sexually active women with natural pubic hair are extinct. The bald eagle fad, originally sparked by young urban women, 24 - 7 internet pornography and seven entrepreneurial Brazilian sisters in the late '80s, has now spread even to married, non-sexually active, non-urban females. And younger male patients now man-scape too. I recently quizzed a group of sexually active male college students – none had ever seen female pubic hair!

And it's not just doctoring in Beverly Hills, the cosmetic epicenter of the world. A recent representative U.S. study confirmed just how widespread the trend is – 75 percent of American adults groom pubic hair (84 percent women, 66 percent men).

Bulletin: Extreme pubic grooming is not a harmless fad.

**Total hair removal increases the risk of genital
herpes virus (HSV) and human papilloma
virus (HPV) by as much as 400 percent!**

Whether you mow pubic hair with razors or shavers, or rip it out by waxing, you wreak havoc on your delicate skin. The outer skin layer (epidermis) — usually a solid barrier — gets lots of little "micro tears," permitting easy access into the body by STD pathogens, especially HPV, HSV, HIV and syphilis that infect by passing directly through genital skin.

Even folks practicing less extreme pubic hair grooming get more STDs than expected. True, on average, groomers have more lifetime sex partners than non-groomers (17 versus 14), but researchers accounting for total number of partners still found STD risk increased dramatically.

Given the broad diversity of clothing, shoes and hairstyles – why the recent below-the-beltline hairless conformity? A quarter of women remove all genital hair at least monthly, another quarter cut or trim at least weekly. Men use electric razors more than women (40 versus 10 percent), while women use non-electric razors more than men (60 versus 35 percent). Others prefer waxing. Why do some women and even men go through the pain of regularly waxing? (Don't laugh. I guarantee men wax. I've seen several cases of ball waxing gone bad.)

Peer pressure, aesthetics and hygiene are reasons given for going thru the self-inflicted pain of waxing. We all conform to peer pressure. God forbid any girl sitting poolside dares risk exposing even one pubic hair. But it's hygiene — the most common reason women give for extreme grooming — that has me flummoxed.

It's logical: No pubic hair means less retained sweat, less trapped dead skin, less dirt, less smells, less skin bacteria... overall cleaner. Right? Wrong!

**Radical pubic grooming does not make
your lady garden more hygienic.
*This is a myth.***

The entire medical profession got sucked into this rabbit hole in the '80s and '90s. Back then, surgical patients had their operative site completely shaved to help sterilize the site. But then a funny thing happened. Studies emerged in the late 1990s revealing the age-old pre-operative shaving ritual paradoxically increased infections! Shaving caused microscopic breaks in the skin, which gave nasty pathogens a toehold. PS: Surgeons trying to minimize post-operative infections no longer shave their patients pre-operatively.

Pubic hair is no evolutionary screw-up; It signals, cushions, protects and entices. Pubic hair signals exactly when the body is green lit for reproduction. Pubic hair cushions sexual contact and limits "trauma"— friction scrapes on fragile genital skin. Pubic hair follicles entice by adding extra sensory pleasure and secreting pheromones, a legitimate aphrodisiac scent. Hair lets these sexy pheromones stick around longer.

So, as you tweeze, shave, wax, laser or Nair away genital hair, be aware. There are repercussions!

1. You remove natural protection and sex appeal.
2. You cause microscopic abrasions along with occasional overt cuts and scrapes.
3. You allow easy access for fungus, bacteria and viruses adept at skin-to-skin contagion, especially resistant staph (MRSA), syphilis, genital herpes, HIV, HPV and molluscum contagiosum (tiny nuisance skin warts cause by a pox virus that can be spread sexually).
4. You cause itchiness as the skin heals. Itching leads to scratching. Scratching leads to further micro abrasions. Which causes more itching... and susceptibility to infection.

There are many different grooming options. Electric shavers are simple and inexpensive but not adept at conforming to the unique pubic skin types and contours. Razor blades — after considerable practice — yield superior results. Still, slicing across irregular labial lip crevices is generally a losing bet. And to keep smooth, you've got to shave at least twice a week. Your skin takes at least two days to heal. Hummm. That doesn't leave a lot of safe play time.

Wax option: Expensive, painful and time consuming. Side effects include occasionally spreading infections via contaminated scissors, tweezers, or improperly sterilized surfaces. The worst of esthetician faux-pas: using the same spatula on multiple clients ("double dipping") in poorly run professional salons. Double dipping holds the bacteria in the wax where it can lead to infections in subsequent unknowing clients. Another possible problem is that the wax can literally fry the fragile labial lips, causing additional discomfort, rash and STD risk.

Electrolysis option: Electrolysis is permanent hair removal. Multiple sessions with an electronically charged needle zaps the hair root and kills the hair follicle. It hurts, there's no guarantee that every last hair is eradicated and it's expensive. But, long term, repetitive genital trauma is avoided. Downside: If pubic hair comes back in fashion, you are out of luck.

Depilatory option: Depilatories are strong bases (like bleach) that break hair bonds allowing unwanted hair to slough off. Skin is also damaged by these chemicals but after healing, it stays smooth days longer than shaving as the hair is detached lower down the hair shaft. Depilatories are a quick, less masochistic, less painful and less costly way to bare skin. But beware. These strong alkaline chemicals can burn delicate vagina, urethra and perianal mucous membranes.

Laser option: Laser is a very powerful energy source. An inexperienced operator can burn, pigment or permanently scar your skin. Done properly, the laser vaporizes the hair root. This causes small plumes of smoke that have a sulfur-like smell. Laser pulses feel like warm pinpricks or a rubber band being snapped against the skin. Most patients need up to six laser treatments on a monthly basis and remain hair-free for months although maintenance treatments are usually needed. If hair does regrow, it's less noticeable. In the past, only people with light skin could safely have laser hair removal. Today, laser hair removal is a treatment option for patients with dark skin too.

Waxing, depilatories and especially electrolysis and laser hair removal are superior to shaving in terms of STD risk. While all treatments damage skin, the former options need fewer repeat maintenance treatments.

There is an extreme groomer silver lining! In the 1980s, I'd be called on a daily basis to search through pubic hair for tiny pencil tip sized moving pubic lice or their annoyingly minute white eggs. Lice need course pubic hair for their eggs to latch onto allowing the full reproduction cycle. When there is no pubic hair, pubic lice cannot survive.

DOCTOR H'S OBSERVATION:

**The natural habitat of pubic
lice has been destroyed. They are now an
endangered species. I haven't seen one in years!**

Doctors H and K Recommend:
1. Consider going retro with a full '70s bush or shaving or waxing less — i.e. a landing strip.
2. Always use clean, fresh, and sharp razors.
3. Shave in the direction of hair growth, this helps prevent nicks and ingrown hairs
4. Shave smart! If men shaved beards the way women shave labia, men's faces would be all scarred up.
5. Treat irritated or red skin with gentle anti-bacterial soap or cleansers.
6. Only book professional licensed estheticians who follow sterile techniques with obsessive-compulsive fervor (i.e. soaking tools in hospital-grade disinfectant between procedures).
7. Remember fads are temporary. But if you really believe Barbie doll genitals is an enduring goal, consider permanent hair removal (laser treatments or electrolysis).
8. If you have an active STD, especially HSV outbreaks or HPV warts, don't play with fire. Cutting into infected skin can augment infectivity to yourself (local spread) and to others.
9. Extreme grooming is associated with four times the risk of some STDs that gain entrance through damaged skin — specially HPV and HSV – while lowering pubic lice infestations. Condoms work far better when your genital skin is entirely intact.
10. Wait 48 hours after hair removal before engaging in sex.

CHAPTER 9
Hepatitis A, B and C:
Common Viruses that Can Ravage Your Liver

In early 1995, I'd just finished a lecture to a National Hockey League Group in San Francisco, when I got a real shock. Moments after stepping into a hotel bathroom, I noticed I had the strangest deep fluorescent orange pee!

I racked my brain, WTF? I felt perfectly fine. I had done an intense 5-mile wharf run that morning but didn't feel dehydrated (concentrated urine can be a dark yellow) or sore (massive muscle breakdown turns urine tea colored). Hepatitis colors urine brown and I had absolutely no hepatitis risks (no foreign travel, no transfusions, no needle sticks, no questionable eating locales, little if any booze and I was in a long term monogamous relationship). I took no vitamins, the number one cause of funky urine tints. I hadn't had rhubarb, beets or other obvious urine coloring foods. Was it some Chinatown delicacy I'd eaten?

I awoke the next morning back in Los Angeles feeling like Sampson with no hair. I gasped out of breath after jogging just one block alongside my daughter as she practiced balancing on her new bike. I staggered back home, and while shaving for work, I belatedly made a self-diagnosis. The whites of my eyes were ever so slightly yellowed. I had freaking hepatitis!

I got an instant pang of anxiety because I remembered several other doctors whose careers were derailed after getting persistent Hep B from work related accidental needle sticks. I was also upset every textbook description of hepatitis claimed the urine turned brown, not the fluorescent orange I was experiencing! My face was now yellower than my painted-with-betadine wrestling days. I was nauseated, beat tired and achy. But worse by far was the non-stop total body itch. For the first time in my life, I had to stay home from work. Lab tests later that day indeed revealed liver tests off the charts. Several

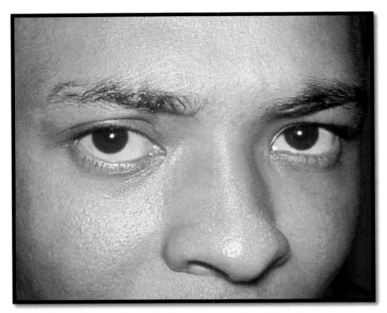

Figure 13 - Yellowed (jaundiced) skin and yellow (icteric) eyes

days later, I finally got good news. The hepatitis antibody tests confirmed I had acute Hep A, not the more ominous Hep B or C.

People usually get hepatitis A from contaminated food or water. I was no exception. A little detective work found that exactly 6 weeks before my crazy colored urine, I had shared a lunch with an employee who in retrospect had an undiagnosed case of mild Hep A: a transient low-level headache, fever and fatigue.

Hepatitis A can also be spread through sex. An infectious virus can be found for weeks in saliva, urine and stool. My wife got an immediate gamma globulin shot to lower her risk. Fortunately, she never got my illness.

Here's the you-can't-make-this-stuff-up weird coincidence – just days later the Hepatitis A vaccine was officially released!

Over the last 20 years, the Hep A vaccine has proven to be highly effective and safe. It's required for school entry in 43 states, California being one of the seven outliers. Just recently, California experienced the largest outbreak of hepatitis A in 25 years, including a few dozen deaths, directly related to that arcane vaccine policy. Did California do anything to update it? Noooooo.

Take it from me, you don't want to get Hep A. Make sure you're vaccinated, especially if you travel. And for goodness sake, get your kids vaccinated. Remember, there were several dozen deaths from the 2017 Hep A epidemic in

California referenced above. Yes, vaccination can be uncomfortable for a day or two, but the balance of benefits to risks is far on the side of benefits. For the sake of our own, and the public's health, we must push sound vaccination policy including routine vaccination for school entry. Let parents whose children have medical reasons not to get vaccinated, obtain a medical exemption.

Bottom line, since the vaccine was licensed, Hep A has dropped from 31,000 to fewer than 1,500 cases per year in the U.S.

Hepatitis B: The More Ominous Hepatitis

Whereas severe hepatitis and death is unusual for Hep A, the Hep B virus commonly kills.

If acquired at childbirth from an infected mother, Hep B becomes a lifelong persistent infection leading to cirrhosis, liver cancer and premature death. If Hep B is acquired in adulthood, usually via sex, it causes a "hepatitis" attack with jaundice 3-6 months after contact. Five percent then go on to persistent infection and resultant cirrhosis, liver cancer and premature death. There is no cure for individuals with persistent Hep B, however, just recently, excellent treatments have been discovered. These anti-Hep B medicines have to be taken for life – similar to the lifelong anti-viral treatments needed to control HIV.

Hep B is spread via sex, blood exposure and childbirth just like HIV, but Hep B is ten-fold more contagious. Condoms work very well to prevent Hep B sexual transmission, but again, the best protection is vaccination. It's even possible to vaccinate a newborn to totally prevent transmission from a mother with persistent Hep B (four doses of Hep B vaccine beginning with a first dose just hours after birth).

The 99 percent effective and safe hepatitis B vaccine arrived on the scene in 1991. With widespread vaccination in the U.S. (it's a routine childhood immunization AND required for school entry in every state) and in many parts of the world - hepatitis B infections, liver cancer and premature deaths have dropped precipitously.

In the U.S., 19,000 new Hep B infections occur yearly. Immigration from countries not requiring infant vaccination is resulting in more Americans (422,000) living with persistent Hep B infection. In poor countries, 1 percent of newborns are infected at birth and over a quarter of a million persons eventually die prematurely due to persistent Hep B. Currently, about 260 million people worldwide have chronic Hep B infection; 25 - 40 percent will go

---

on to develop fatal cirrhosis or liver cancer if treatment is not provided – worse case resulting in 786,000 deaths each year.

In the last several decades, more than 1 billion doses of Hep B vaccine have been administered worldwide — mostly to infants. I'm going to repeat myself here, because their are so many vaccine naysayers, you rarely hear about the documented prevention powers of vaccines anymore. In Taiwan, a country where more than 15 percent of children previously got Hep B, universal vaccination programs begun 25 years ago have lowered that number to now less than 1 percent of children. More importantly, the number of Hep B associated liver cancers in young adults has dropped by a similar amount.

Based just on the intensive worldwide Hep B vaccine push from 2000-2011, an astronomical *3.7 million deaths* have been prevented.

Dr. K was a medical intern in Bellevue hospital in 1991 and one of the first in line to get the newly developed hepatitis B vaccine. That was a godsend in the setting of a packed public New York City hospital, where fulminant (you are going to die soon) hepatitis B was an everyday diagnosis. Here's the rub: one errant needle stick from a hepatitis B patient and you had a 1 in 3 chance of contracting infectious Hep B (not to mention a chance getting HIV too). Unlike today, where teams of highly skilled phlebotomists and nurses collect blood and insert IV's, back then it was the job of exhausted, overworked interns to do it all. Dr. K's experience was similar to mine – it wasn't unusual to suffer a needle stick or exposure of some sort every month or so.

It was a dangerous game of *blood exposure* Russian roulette.

Hepatitis C: The Most Ominous Hepatitis

Hep C is by far the most ominous hepatitis virus. Like Hep A and Hep B, it can acutely infect the liver causing exhaustion, jaundice (yellowing of the eyes and skin) and itchiness. But if you get Hep C as an adult, the future is much scarier. Whereas only 1 and 5 percent of new adult infections with Hep A and Hep B respectively go on to potentially disastrous persistent infections (the rest self-heal), fully 50 percent of new Hep C infections remain persistent, resulting decades later in cirrhosis, liver cancer and premature death. Partly due to this, and partly due to the success of Hep B vaccination, Hep C has replaced Hep B as the number one cause of liver cancer and liver transplantation in the U.S.

There was widespread transmission of Hep C in the 1950s and 1960s in the United States due to contaminated blood products (transfusions) and contaminated reused needles for injections. The CDC recommends all persons born in the 50s and 60s ("baby boomers") get tested. I remember when getting childhood vaccinations, my pediatrician, a cigarette hanging out of his mouth, pulled out a metal tray of glass hypodermic syringes and reusable needles. The smell of alcohol disinfectant suggested they were sterile, but who knows?

Like Hep B, Hep C can be spread via sex, blood exposure and childbirth. Currently, 2 percent of "baby boomers" are infected with Hep C. About half these past infections have spontaneously cleared and require no further treatment. The remaining infections are "persistent" and require treatment if cirrhosis, liver cancer and premature death are to be averted.

Today, Hep C transmission is almost solely among intravenous drug users who share needles. Hep C is present in semen but except for highly sexually active MSM, sexual transmission is rare. In fact, discordant (one partner has Hep C, the other partner is negative for Hep C) heterosexual couples pass it less than 1 percent per year; the CDC feels this risk is so low, they don't even recommend routine condom use if the couple is otherwise monogamous.

Call me a worrier, but to me, a 1 percent risk of getting Hep C is too high. Testing for Hep C and curing the disease in as little as 8 weeks – we have incredible new anti-viral cocktails, see below – is the best way to remove the admittedly low-risk of getting Hep C sexually.

Curative Treatment: Unlike other chronic viral infections like Hep B, HIV, HPV or HSV, there are complete cures for persistent Hep C! One hundred percent, its gone. No more virus, no more risk for ongoing liver disease, liver cancer or liver transplants. Here are the Hep C cures:

Harvoni (sofosbuvir and ledipasvir): one pill per day X 8 - 12 weeks or
Vosevi (sofosbuvir/velpatasvir/voxilaprevir): one pill per day X 8 weeks or
Mavyret (glecaprevir and pibrentasvir): one pill per day X 8 weeks.

Just last year at UCLA, hepatitis C dropped down to the number two reason for liver transplant. The only way to know if you have hepatitis C is to get the highly accurate blood tests (or oral fluid test in Europe). The first test is a screening antibody test. If it's positive, a follow-up hepatitis C viral RNA test is needed to see if the infection has "self-healed" or became "persistent."

Test/ Interpretation	Hep C antibody screening test	Hep C viral RNA test
Never infected.	(-)	Not applicable
Prior infection but self-healed (50%). **No treatment needed.**	(+)	(-)
Persistent infection, potentially fatal (50%). **Treatment needed.**	(+)	(+)

Table 7: How to Interpret Your Hep C Blood Tests

Always ask your doctor questions. Remember it's the informed consumer in medicine these days that gets the best care.

Doctors do not always do what's right – and that's advice from 2 doctors with combined medical experience of over 60 years.

DOCTORS H AND K RECOMMEND:

Hep A vaccine series routinely in all childhood vaccines

Hep B vaccine series routinely in all childhood vaccines

Hep B vaccine series for unvaccinated persons (i.e. those born before 1992) at high-risk:
- MSM
- IV recreational drug users
- Condom-less sex with individuals born in countries with a high burden of HIV
- Hep C carriers

Hepatitis C test:
- those born in the 1950s or 1960s
- MSM
- IV drug users

CHAPTER 10
Ebola and Zika: Lethal New Viral STDs

Ebola and Zika are the two very recent — and very feared — additions to the "STD's in the U.S." list. While those viruses can be spread through sexual intercourse (up to 30 days after Zika infection and perhaps up to 6 months among survivors with Ebola infection), like Hep C, their predominant route of transmission is not sex.

Ebola is a lethal terror. It spreads like we originally feared HIV might spread.

Specifically, in 1981 we feared the still unnamed HIV virus might:
1. Be uncannily contagious
2. Be spread via tears, sweat and saliva in addition to blood
3. Put family and friends with just casual contact at exceptional high-risk
4. Put health care personal at exceptional high-risk (remember many of us in the early 80s wondered out loud if the hospital should be furnishing us with hazmat suits)
5. Necessitate quarantines of suspected patients, family and exposed health care workers

As it turned out, HIV had *none* of these features. But Ebola:
1. Is uncannily contagious
2. Is spread via tears, sweat and saliva in addition to blood
3. Commonly infects family and friends with just casual contact
4. Commonly infects health care personal (doctors and nurses currently are instructed to wear hazmat suits)
5. Necessitates quarantines of suspected patients, family and exposed health care workers (remember Dr. Nancy Synderman, NBC's medical correspondent, who admitted she violated Ebola quarantine mandates in 2015)

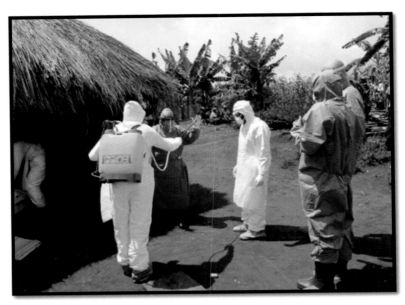

Figure 14 - Health care workers attending "decontamination rounds" outside a rural african ebola hospital (CDC Ebola Website)

Zika is a ticking time bomb for pregnant women living in Zika endemic regions like Brazil. The Zika infection, spread through a mosquito bite (like malaria), is initially no big deal, with merely flu-like symptoms. But this otherwise innocuous virus can cause devastating fetal deformities which might not be detected until childbirth – leaving expectant families to live in fear.

Both Ebola and Zika virus have been detected in semen and in vaginal fluids. Only male-to-female sexual transmission has been documented for both viruses (and male-to-male for Zika). But although sexual transmission is possible, the chance it actually happens is quite rare. Less than one in a thousand of all Ebola or Zika cases happen through sexual contact.

Ebola is deadly. More than half of all people who get Ebola infection die within a few weeks. Zika is not deadly initially, it's the later pregnancy complications that can be lethal. Thousands of new born babies worldwide die or have lifelong neurologic damage as a result of the congenital Zika infection.

Why is Ebola — far more contagious and deadly than HIV — so much less a threat to world health? Because Ebola sickens then kills its victims so quickly, persons with Ebola have very little time to spread the Ebola virus. Compare that to HIV, where people can have infectious HIV, not know it, yet spread it for 20 or more years. In that regard Ebola is not a very good virus at keeping itself circulating among humans.

Ebola is only able to remain a human threat because it is good at infecting certain kinds of rain forest bats. These bats don't get sick, instead they keep the virus circulating by spreading Ebola to other bats and other animals. When a human sustains an infected bat bite or comes into contact with infected bush meat, the virus enters the body, multiplies quickly and stimulates the immune system to release toxins in the blood stream. Without supportive care, those toxins often kill that person within days.

The protracted West African Ebola outbreaks were enabled by a century old tradition: cleaning and bathing recently deceased relatives. Since Ebola virus survives in body fluids at room temperature for days — some family members adhering to those long-standing customs get infected — and the cycle of transmission continues.

Zika on the other hand, because it is mosquito born and exists in a steady state in animals like monkeys and apes, tends to impact thousands or more when it enters a population that has not been exposed to Zika before. Nearly everyone who goes outside and suffers a mosquito bite will be infected. Once infected however, you gain immunity and cannot get Zika a second time.

How many are currently infected (Ebola and Zika prevalence)?

Ebola manifests itself in outbreaks, sudden increases in a small geographically isolated population. The largest reported outbreak of Ebola — more than 25,000 cases — occurred in Western Africa in 2014 - 2015. The 2017 outbreak was much smaller – 10 cases. The most recent 2018 outbreak in the Democratic Republic of the Congo has infected over 55 persons, killing half of them.

The frequency of Zika infection in different areas of the world ranges from 0 to 10 - 20 percent. In the United States, Zika infection is very rare, estimated at less than 0.1 percent.

How many get new infections each year (incidence)?

New Ebola cases range from none a year for several years to thousands in a given year globally. In the United States there were 2 locally acquired and 7 additional cases during the 2015 outbreak among doctors or nurses returning from West Africa. Eight of those 9 cases survived. The one patient that did die was misdiagnosed and turned away from the hospital on his first visit to the emergency room.

New Zika cases in the U.S. range from none to a few dozen per year depending on travel. More than 3,000 babies were born with serious deformities and neurological complications in the recent 2015 - 2016 Brazilian Zika outbreak. Travelers to regions of the world where Zika has been reported (French Polynesia, Brazil, Puerto Rico and the Caribbean), in theory, could still be at risk, but since 2016 new cases seem to be unusual.

Ebola and Zika: How do you get it?

Ebola is acquired by direct skin or mucous membrane (eyes, mouth) contact with blood-contaminated body fluids. Ebola can live outside the body on countertops, doorknobs and toilet seats for several hours but can survive in a drop of blood at room temp for several days. Sexual transmission, while possible with male Ebola survivors for up to 6 months, is rare.

Zika is spread through mosquitos. An infected mosquito secretes Zika virus during a mosquito bite. Zika virus DNA has been detected in male semen up to 9 months after infection but essentially all sexual transmission occurs in the first month after infection. Relatively few cases of male-to-female and male-to-male Zika transmission have been documented while no female to male cases have been reported. Zika has been detected in vaginal secretions but perhaps the amount of virus is too low to allow transmission.

Ebola and Zika: First Warning Signs

Ebola will make you sick. Most people with Ebola have a high fever, fatigue, joint and muscle aches, like a knock-out flu. Ebola can progress to sepsis — very low blood pressure, internal bleeding and death. About 50 percent of those who get Ebola will die in a few weeks. In the United States, with prompt top level ICU care, a far higher percent of patients will survive.

Most often people bitten by a Zika infected mosquito develop no symptoms. Some however, get fever, vague flu feelings and a skin rash. The fever and rash will go away in about 1 - 2 weeks. The most serious Zika complication occurs in infected pregnant woman, 20 - 50 percent of whom will transmit Zika virus to the unborn fetus resulting in miscarriage, preterm birth or babies born with serious birth defects like micro encephalopathy (very small heads). Those babies may die within the first few months or live with long term neurological and developmental defects.

Zika might even be causing problems for babies that seemed fine at birth. Scientists are just now beginning to figure out more long-ranging effects of Zika. A study involving 1,450 babies exposed to the virus found that 6 percent were born with birth defects, and an additional 14 percent developed problems that could be attributed to the virus by the time they turned one.

Ebola and Zika: Natural History if You Don't Treat

Like many viruses, there is no specific antiviral treatment for either Ebola or Zika infections. About 50 percent of those who get Ebola will initially be violently ill and quickly die (much better odds if you have access to a top-notch western medicine ICU).

Most persons infected with Zika are asymptomatic and unaware that they ever got it.

Ebola and Zika: How to Diagnosis

If you have high fever, weakness, excessive bleeding and have had recent contact with an Ebola patient – get to the nearest ICU. You may have Ebola.

For less obvious situations, an Ebola virus DNA test is now available which turns positive just a few days after exposure. The usual period between exposure and illness is about 1 week.

There is no reason to even try to diagnose Zika in a female if she is not pregnant or not planning on getting pregnant in the next year. There is no reason to even try to diagnose Zika in a male if when with women of child bearing age, he always uses a condom.

If a woman contemplating pregnancy or already pregnant lives or travels in a Zika endemic region (i.e. Brazil), regardless of symptoms, she should get a Zika blood antibody test. Most tests will become positive about 3 - 4 weeks after exposure. The tests are generally accurate but sometimes other viruses like Dengue or Chikungungwa can cause false-positive tests. Be sure your doctor knows what test he or she is doing! If positive, pregnancy should be delayed for 6 months, or if already pregnant, the fetus should be evaluated by a specialized ultrasound. If the male partner of a pregnant woman travels in a Zika endemic region (i.e. Brazil), a Zika blood test is optional because even if the test is negative, he should not have sex without a condom for at least 1 - 6 months from the time of mosquito bites.

Ebola and Zika: Are They Curable?

No. If you survive Ebola, you may be protected from future infection. Most Zika infections are asymptomatic, and there is no cure but infection is of short duration. The body's immune system completely clears the infection and immunity eventually develops - preventing reinfection.

Ebola and Zika: Are They Treatable?

Yes, most persons in highly developed settings can "weather the Ebola storm" with state of the art ICU care, specifically replenishment of blood products, dialysis and IV meds to thwart low blood pressure. Unfortunately, Ebola hot spots like West Africa have few hospitals and even fewer modern ICUs. While there is no medicine to specifically treat Zika, almost all adults clear the infection on their own and develop immunity to future infection. There are no medicines currently available to treat infants born to mothers with Zika infection.

Ebola and Zika: Infectivity

In the United States, nearly zero. Both infections are very rare and almost always acquired in travelers to areas of the world where outbreaks are occurring. Sexual transmission of Zika may rarely occur from a recent traveler to a sex partner through condom-less sex. Women who want to become pregnant (or are pregnant) should refrain from having sex without a condom with a man who has visited areas with ongoing Zika transmission for at least 3 months from his return.

Women (or men) should not have sex without a condom with an Ebola survivor for at least 6 months after his initial illness.

Ebola and Zika: Prevention

a. *Awareness is prevention:* Know the facts: Although very rare, condom-less sex with a recent traveler to a place where there is an ongoing Zika or Ebola epidemic can lead to infection.

b. *Prophylaxis is prevention:* Avoiding contact with Ebola infectious blood or blood-tinged body fluids or using mosquito repellent and wearing long sleeves and pants (for Zika) are the best ways to prevent infection.

c. *Protection is prevention:* Condoms – Latex (or polyurethane) male or female condoms work. Condoms serve as barriers to the spread of viruses and bacteria so they can easily hold or block viruses like Ebola or Zika. However, for condoms to work, they must be correctly used. (See video on how to use a male condom by Planned Parenthood).

d. *Vaccination:* There is a highly promising Ebola virus vaccine. Preliminary data has shown the experimental vaccine (VSV-EBOV) to be highly effective and it is currently being tested in at risk individuals in the 2018 Ebola outbreak in the Democratic Republic of the Congo.

CHAPTER 11
Genital Herpes: The Elephant in America's Bedroom

Genital herpes is the quintessential elephant in America's bedroom.

The majority of persons who have genital herpes are completely unaware. The minority who are aware are rarely if ever brave enough to acknowledge their herpes diagnosis: not lovers, not family members, not applicants to dating shows, not movie actors doing nude scenes with random co-stars, not politicians, not judges — not even doctors. And who can blame them? Herpes is a secret STD with a blistering stigma fueled by fear and ignorance. As proof, look no further than ABC's long-running *Bachelor* reality show. If an applicant tests positive for genital herpes, they are summarily disqualified from participating in the show and told to "see a doctor."

Because genital herpes is never discussed, you assume it's relatively uncommon. *Wrong.*

Because you've never had a visible lesion, you assume there's no way you have herpes. *Wrong.*

Because you get regular STD checks, you assume you've been tested and do not have herpes. *Wrong.*

Because of the intense social shame and the frequent hyperbolic response when you reveal the herpes diagnosis to a partner, you assume, except for HIV, herpes is medically more dangerous than all other STD's. *Wrong again.*

Recurrent herpes lesions have been popping out on human genital skin for thousands of years. Scholars named the disease herpes (in Greek this means *to creep or crawl*) after observing how the rash slowly expands over a period of several days. But throughout human history, no one paid herpes much attention —unlike gonorrhea and syphilis which were the basis for huge disease control campaigns, especially during World Wars I and II. Herpes, on the other hand, was no big deal. The rash was transient. The symptoms were mild. Sometimes "cold" sores popped out on the edge of the lip or under the nose. Sometimes the "cold" sores appeared on the genitals. Who cared? No one! Want proof?

To illustrate how herpes was stigma-free in the recent past, let's go back to London in 1975, a year when best estimates are that over 70 percent of the population had herpes infections of one type or another. 1975 was also the year a British psychiatrist wrote a famous medical paper titled *"Psychological morbidity in a clinic for STDs."* He interviewed 100 patients at an urban STD clinic and found 45 had significant anxiety due to concerns about a new STD. However, despite many documented cases of HPV, crabs, chlamydia, gonorrhea, trichomonas and yeast – *not one of these 100 individuals complained of or were diagnosed with herpes!* Not even one speck of herpes angst!

Suddenly, in the late 1970s, at the height of the sexual revolution, this laid-back attitude inexplicably spun 180 degrees.

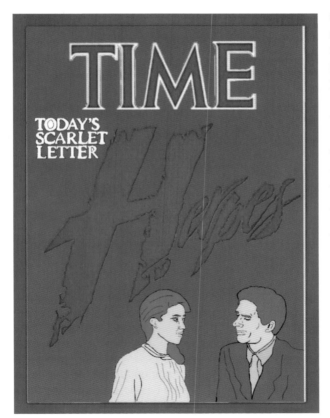

One theory: Biomedical research foundation Burroughs Wellcome had a new drug called Zovirax that worked well in suppressing herpes but there wasn't much of a market for their drug. So, they ran clever direct-to-consumer ads exploiting the difference between good herpes "type 1" and bad herpes "type 2." Voila! Free sex might have undesirable side effects!

A villain was born.

A second theory: Irresponsible journalism. This representation of the August 2, 1982 Time magazine cover is exhibit #1.

Figure 15 – An artist's rendering of the gaudy 'Scarlet Letter' herpes cover, August 2, 1982

The *Time* magazine cover story was a below-the-belt

STD nuclear blast: It detailed recurrent painful genital herpes attacks, wildfire contagiousness, childbirth disasters and incurability.

> "After chastity slouched off into exile in the '60s, the sexual revolution encountered little resistance. Indeed, in the age of the Pill, Penthouse Pets and porn-movie cassettes, the revolution looked so sturdily permanent that sex seemed to subside into a simple consumer item.
>
> Now, suddenly, the old fears and doubts are edging back. So is the fire and brimstone rhetoric of the Age of Guilt. The reason for all this dolor: herpes, an ancient viral infection that can be transmitted during sex, recurs fitfully and cannot be treated or cured."

Time magazine, 8/2/1982

The gaudy *Scarlet Letter Herpes* cover — and the breathless commentary — thrust herpes center stage and marked the high (or low) point in American's full-frontal herpes hysteria.

The message was clear. At all costs, avoid having sex with someone with herpes.

Overnight, herpes became the country's most loathed disease.

Infection vs. Disease

Ironically, in most cases herpes isn't really even a disease!

When someone has an infection and doesn't know it, or that infection doesn't make one sick, generally, doctors do not say that person has a "disease." A "disease" is a condition that causes symptoms and/or over the long-term causes sickness. Since people can have HSV1 or HSV2 infection and not be sick, those people have what we call "silent infection" or just "infection."

Genital herpes causes only infection in most, and disease in the minority of cases. We don't exactly know just why that is – we do know that a weakened immune system predisposes to sickness and disease.

Herpes: Two Types, Two Scenarios

Herpes viruses are everywhere – in every age group, every country and every ethnicity. There are at least 8 different human herpes viruses that cause disease. The most notable are chickenpox, shingles, mononucleosis, roseola (a toddler disease with high fever, rash and occasional seizures), Kaposi's sarcoma and oral and genital herpes.

In common parlance, when people talk about *herpes*, they're referring to herpes simplex virus 2 (HSV2), which most call "genital herpes" or "the bad type." This virus mostly remains silent in a group of nerve cells located in the lower spine but occasionally HSV2 manifests as tiny irritations or clusters of sensitive blisters in the genital, buttock or peri-anal regions.

Herpes simplex type 1 (HSV1) also mostly remains silent, residing undetected in a group of nerve cells near the ear. A first-time symptomatic viral infection can show up anywhere on the face, lips, mouth or even on the tonsils simulating severe strep throat. Remember though, HSV1 can switch hit, it also frequently shows up in the genital/buttock/peri-anal regions.

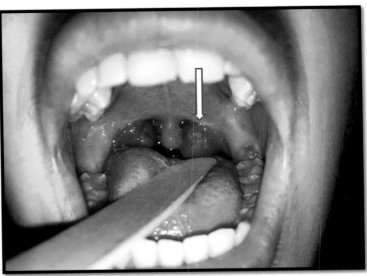

Figure 16 - Initial HSV1 showing up as swelling and painful sores (arrow) on the tonsil in an adult woman

Subsequently, HSV1 may recur, typically showing up every several months on the outer lip as small, round, superficial blisters that soon break, leaving open sores. Herpes blisters near the eyes or in or around the nose are less typical. These facial outbreaks are called "cold sores," "fever blisters" or the "good type."

How many Americans have Herpes type 1?

Each year, *1.6 million* American adults will catch HSV1 – 1.2 million genitally and 400,000 orally. Women are 10 to 15 percent more likely than men to be infected as adults.

Currently, *127 million* Americans have HSV1. Approximately 67 million got infected as children. 60 million got infected as adults — 35 million with oral

HSV1 (primarily kissing) and 25 million with genital HSV1 (oral sex). Estimates are that 80 plus percent of Americans older than 70 have HSV1.

In the past, HSV1 was essentially only a childhood disease. Nowadays, *1.6 million* American children still catch HSV1 (not an STD) – all orally, often in the first few years of life, when an actively infectious (but unaware) relative plants a loving kiss.

Two decades ago, nearly all the children in low income countries and half of all children in high income countries like the U.S. got HSV1. Now, in America, only about one-quarter of children get HSV1, presumably due to heightened awareness on the part of cold-sore-infected parents and grandparents. Ironically, this heightened vigilance on the part of doting family members coupled with the generations-old mistaken belief oral sex is completely safe – has spawned an alarming new STD epidemic! But more on that later.

How many Americans have Herpes type 2?

Each year, about *1.4 million* American adults will catch HSV2, essentially all genital as HSV2 rarely if ever shows up orally.

Currently, *30 million* Americans have HSV2.

On average, 8 and 16 percent of adult men and women, respectively, aged 16 - 49 currently have HSV2. Estimates are that 30 percent of Americans older than 70 have HSV2.

Herpes simplex virus 2, like HSV1, has also become less common over the last several decades. In 2000, 12 and 24 percent of 16 - 49-year-old men and women, respectively, had HSV2.

Women are twice as likely as men to be infected with HSV2 because of anatomic differences that make it easier for the female genitalia to get infected. Rates of HSV2 infection also vary widely by ethnicity and geographical region (higher in the Southeast, especially urban areas) and higher among men who have sex with men (about 22 percent).

The HSV Paradox

Genital herpes infection is benign. It does not cause cancer. It does not cause infertility. It does not cause internal organ damage or early death. Still, genital herpes is dreaded on par with a life-threatening disease (which it is not).

While persons with STDs often get transient "self-doubt" or "less-of-a-person" depression, those with a herpes diagnosis get a triple dose of guilt, humiliation and fear — sometimes requiring professional counseling. (When that happens, their infection has become a "stigma-inflicted" disease). Occasionally their herpes infections cause transient symptoms like sores or discomfort. While not considered serious by doctors, patients do feel like they have a disease.

When internet STD site discussions turn to recently contracted genital herpes, not infrequently, suicidal ideation is expressed. I'll never forget a patient so distraught after contracting herpes that institutionalization was required to avert her sworn plan: speeding off a local bridge to end her misery.

Some of this over the top reaction to herpes moderated in the 90's – by comparison to HIV, herpes no longer seemed so horrible. Still, while it became somewhat permissible in the late 90's for individuals to admit in pubic they were infected with HIV — or serious human herpes viruses like shingles, mononucleosis, cytomegalovirus or even cancer-causing Kaposi's sarcoma virus — no one was openly admitting to genital herpes infections.

The best way to eliminate stigma is by shining a light on the facts:

- Unlike HIV, Hep B, Hep C and HPV – herpes doesn't kill or cause serious physical disease.
- Unlike gonorrhea, chlamydia, and mycoplasma – herpes doesn't make you infertile.
- Unlike syphilis – herpes left unattended doesn't slowly cannibalize your body from the inside out, making you crazy or blind.
- Unlike pubic lice – HSV is wimpy. It can't live outside the human body for more than a few seconds. It doesn't spread from dirty towels or toilet seats.

Yes, both HSV1 and HSV2 infections can be a real nuisance. But in 99 percent of cases, symptoms are minor or nonexistent.

However, in today's America, if you test positive for HSV2, you're a leper! You must be low class. You must be "dirty." You must be promiscuous. In truth, half of genital herpes sufferers have had four or fewer lifetime sex partners. Hardly immoral by any standard.

In America today, if you test positive for HSV2, your sex life is screwed. Ethically you need to disclose your status to each new partner, and with no education or insight into the baseless stigma, you fear (for good reason) your partner might just bolt for the bedroom door.

So, what do those aware of their herpes positive status say when contemplating sex? Mostly nothing. Eighty-plus percent decline to share their herpes diagnosis with new partners.

The majority of persons who have genital herpes are completely unaware. The minority who are aware are rarely if ever brave enough to acknowledge their herpes diagnosis.

How bad is genital herpes stigma?

Every disease has its famous "champions" – celebrities agreeing to publicly acknowledge their or a loved one's disease.

Colon cancer: President Ronald Reagan, Sharon Osbourne, Katie Couric (publicized husband's disease)

Alzheimer's: Nancy Reagan, Burgess Meredith, Glen Campbell

Prostate cancer: Ben Stiller, Robert De Niro, General Colin Powell

Breast cancer: Angelina Jolie, Julia Louis-Dreyfus, Melissa Etheridge

Parkinson's Disease: Mohammed Ali, Michael J. Fox

Hepatitis: Pamela Anderson, Steven Tyler, Jim Nabors, Phil Lesh (founding member of the Grateful Dead)

HPV: Amy Schumer, Ali Wong

HPV: (cervical cancer) Erin Andrews (sportscaster), Marissa Jaret Winokur (Broadway Actress)

HPV: (oral cancer) Michael Douglas, Bruce Dickerson (Iron Maiden singer), Rikki Rockett (Poison drummer)

HPV: (anal cancer) Farrah Fawcett

HIV: Rock Hudson, Magic Johnson, Charlie Sheen

HSV: No one!!!

Despite nearly *160 million* Americans with
herpes, not one celeb has ever publicly stepped
forward and owned a herpes diagnosis!

That of course hasn't stopped the gossip-hungry press (over half of whom personally have herpes as well) from compiling long lists of "rumored" herpes-afflicted celebrities based on civil or divorce depositions, public photographs with suspicious lip sores or leaked anti-herpes pharmacy prescriptions. Understandably, celebs insist on having herpes meds filled under a pseudonym even though the pseudo names can result in legal actions taken against the prescribing doctor. Remember the ugly aftermath of narcotic prescriptions given to Michael Jackson under pseudonyms? So, it's one more emotional tug of war for us prescribing doctors: Should we prescribe according to the letter of the law? Use the celebrity's real name? Or break the law by using a pseudonym or their personal assistant's name – knowing full well the prescription drug represents sensitive information that gossip sites offer money to get.

How did things get this insane?

The *Bachelor* TV show banning potential contestants with "herpes" is the most recent example of villainizing herpes. And why not? This stigmatized STD is an easy punching bag. Errant "old school" medical teachings also feed into today's fear and ignorance.

Allow me to revisit the medical teachings of the '80s and '90s — much of which persist today. Then we'll contrast that with what we know today, illuminating the mistruths drilled into our collective brains over the last few decades. Hopefully, comparing those "old school" ideas to recent knowledge will explain why some doctors, and most patients, remain woefully in the dark.

What to expect when genital HSV strikes: the *"old-school"* teaching.

1) When you contract genital herpes, you know it!
Back when I was in med school, I was taught the first herpes outbreak is painfully obvious - lots of raw bursting blisters often accompanied by fever, swollen groin nodes, burning urination (sometimes with discharge), total body aches and headaches.

2) Genital herpes means lifelong recurrent painful blister outbreaks during which herpes can be spread.
I was also taught recurrent attacks were an inescapable component of herpes. The recurrent outbreaks were milder and more localized than the initial. They'd

occur at similar genital locations heralded by tingling sensations (known as the prodrome) followed a day or two later by a cluster of tiny blisters on a red base erupting somewhere in the penis/vulvar territories. The repeat attacks signaled infectiousness. Responsible persons were told and expected to avoid intercourse from the time they felt prodromal tingling to the time the herpes blisters broke, scabbed, then fully healed — namely when the scabs fell off. Doctors worried herpes sufferers might be contagious a day before the premonitory tingling, but we were told to inform our patients, "You're good to go at all other times."

In 1985, herpes sufferers caught a break: acyclovir, a legit anti-herpes drug, was released. An effective vaccine would have been better, but daily medication, though a pain in the ass to remember, was a step forward. Now anyone with painful outbreaks could medicate the symptoms, and the viral contagion away. More to the point, herpes sufferers who could not bring themselves to level with new partners (i.e., almost everyone with the diagnosis) had an ethical "end-around." They would take acyclovir daily, "preventing" recurrent attacks and presumably eradicating transmission risk. They then could sleep at night despite withholding their infection status from their partner.

Our Understanding of Herpes Suddenly Turned Upside Down

Yikes!!! In the year 2000, a lot of what we doctors "knew" about herpes suddenly went up in a billow of smoke. Key facts I was taught and had preached repeatedly to hundreds and hundreds of patients, turned out to be dead wrong! [An old adage I was taught in Harvard medical school: 50 percent of what we teach you is wrong – unfortunately we do not know which 50 percent!]

Information from two new herpes tests for HSV — Western blot antibody blood testing and PCR viral DNA skin swabs — revolutionized our understanding of herpes.

This game-changer tech:
1) allows accurate diagnosis of herpes infection by an antibody blood test — not just when blisters are present.
2) permits accurate differentiation of HSV1 from HSV2 for the first time by detecting strain specific proteins (PCR viral DNA test) or antibodies (Western blot blood test).
3) allows researchers to observe the exact location, duration and amount of silent herpes shedding — a real-time assessment of contagiousness!

The old way relied on herpes cultures – rubbing a swab over skin, then inoculating the swab on cells in a dish and looking for herpes induced cell death — a hit-or-miss process at best. Contrast this to PCR viral DNA tests, instantly identifying miniature pieces of herpes in any specimen – skin surface, lips, mucous membranes, penis, vagina or vaginal/urethral secretions.

Herpes DNA detection and Western blot antibody blood testing vividly explained why herpes was spreading even when herpes sufferers were acting "responsibly."

What to expect when genital HSV strikes: *the new 2018 reality.*

1) When you first get genital herpes, you know it!

No! That's a myth.

Up to 90 percent feel nothing. Their genital HSV infection begins silently. Several weeks to two months after HSV exposure, the Western blot antibody blood test turns positive. PCR DNA tests of the genitals show intermittent bouts of shedding virus, on average about three days per month. Still the vast majority feel nothing or perhaps something so trivial it's written off as inconsequential intercourse trauma.

This isn't genital HSV infection you say? Unfortunately, it is. Those people are infectious. They sometimes spread herpes to partners.

Some old school teachings do hold true. For instance, 10 percent of those with herpes infection do get discernable symptoms, and the initial attack can sometimes be as painful an ordeal as detailed in the old school section above. Scientists don't yet understand why just that small fraction of herpes cases have symptoms.

When you first get genital herpes, you know it!

**No! That's a myth. Up to 90 percent feel nothing.
Their genital HSV begins silently.**

---

2) Genital herpes means lifelong recurrent painful blister outbreaks during which herpes can be spread.

No! There are several misleading myths here!

Only 5 to 10 percent of those with accurate Western blot proven genital herpes get recurring attacks (i.e. prodromal tingling or shooting sensations to buttock/ legs and/or classic eruptions of genital blisters).

The remaining 90 - 95 percent get no symptoms. Well, not exactly. When those people are fully educated, up to half acknowledge suspicious occurrences! This could be trivial urinary or genital burning, itching, numbness, red bumps, fissures and cracks, or bruising symptoms. These signs of genital herpes may present away from the penis/vulva: out of sight peri-anally or at the original site of the infection (i.e. often penile skin or at the opening of the vagina) or near the nerve endings that reach out from the bottom of the spine, buttocks, or posterior thighs.

Unfortunately, even the half with unequivocal symptom-free genital herpes can transmit herpes. Those individuals silently shed herpes virus 10 percent of the time (about three days per month) thru normal genital skin. It's possible that low levels of virus are only minimally infectious. More studies are needed. But this is an uncomfortable truth. You can get HSV2 or genital HSV1 from a partner who has absolutely never had symptoms or any visible skin findings.

An uncomfortable truth.

You can get HSV2 or genital HSV1 from a partner who has absolutely never had symptoms or any visible skin findings.

For the 5 to 40 percent who get repeat identifiable outbreaks, on average about four times per year, herpes transmission risk is higher immediately prior to and during the outbreaks. This increased transmission risk period averages out to about two days per month. But here's a provocative new research finding: These symptomatic folks also shed virus in between attacks through normal skin — about four days a month. So, in reality, those with discernible recurrent attacks are silently infectious four days and visibly infectious two days, for a total of about six infectious days per month. The old-school doctor recommendation: Don't have intercourse during an attack when risk is high, wait 'til the scabs fall off, then you're OK — is bad advice! It does not take into consideration silent shedding, which is time-wise twice as common as shedding associated with symptomatic lesions.

When anal sex is involved, sores may form inside the rectum resembling ulcerative colitis. If you enjoy anal sex, one of the last taboo topics in medicine, that needs to be openly discussed with your medical care providers.

An oft repeated myth: Herpes is spread by callous HSV-positive infected persons having sex during outbreaks. No! Seventy percent of new herpes cases — well over 1 million — are caused by individuals with no genital symptoms or sores, who don't even know they have herpes! That isn't surprising since symptom-free herpes (infection) is so much more common than symptomatic herpes (disease).

Lastly, let's revisit Acyclovir (and other newer anti-herpes drugs). Can anyone with herpes — especially those with painful outbreaks — medicate the symptoms and the viral contagion away? Anti-herpes drugs at the right dose do reduce symptoms, and in some they may completely suppress transmission risk, but it's nearly impossible to predict who will benefit most. The fact is, on average, those drugs only cut the spread of herpes infection from someone with herpes to someone without herpes by half.

Nirvana? Not so much.

Genital HSV: *How to diagnose in 2018*

1. Visual:
Classic herpes outbreaks: When you see your Aunt Minnie once a year at Thanksgiving, you immediately know it's her. Similarly, a well-trained eye can instantly spot classically appearing groups of small blisters on the penis, labial lips or buttocks regions which strongly suggest a herpes diagnosis. 5 - 10 percent of herpes cases present in this fashion (Figures 17, 18 and 19).

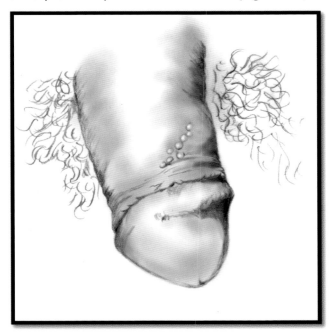

Figure 17 - HSV2. Classic appearing cluster of recurrent herpes blisters on penis

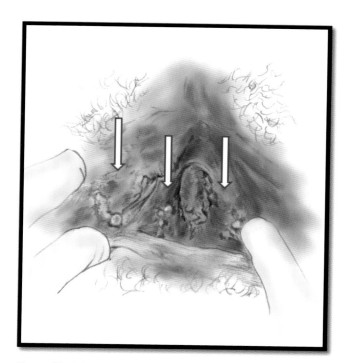

Figure 18 - HSV2. Several clusters of uncomfortable sores on labia (blister tops have come off)

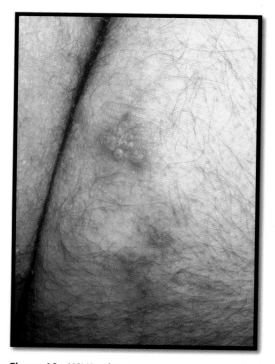

Figure 19 - HSV2. Classic appearing groups of blisters in the upper buttock region (no history of anal sex)

HSV1 vs. HSV2: Is it possible to visually tell the difference between HSV1 and HSV2? No (Figure 20).

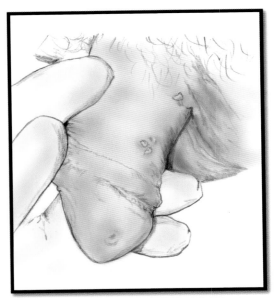

Figure 20 - HSV1. Healing, slightly uncomfortable rash, with blister tops removed leaving multiple open, partially scabbed sores. Blood antibody testing positive for HSV1, negative for HSV2

Atypical herpes outbreaks: The herpes rash and skin complaints may, however, be quite atypical. The rash can be nothing more than an evanescent redness and appear in different locations, like the buttock crease, frustrating an accurate visual diagnosis (Figure 21).

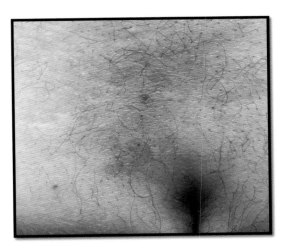

Figure 21 - HSV2. Atypical minor herpes rash on top of buttock (no history of anal intercourse). Western blot antibody testing confirmed this individual had HSV2 infection

Visual diagnosis of herpes is especially difficult in women. Outbreaks can look like nothing more than thin breaks in the skin just inside the vagina or in a fold of the vulva.

Scarring from prior outbreaks: Past herpes outbreaks can leave faint darkened scar tissue (Figure 22).

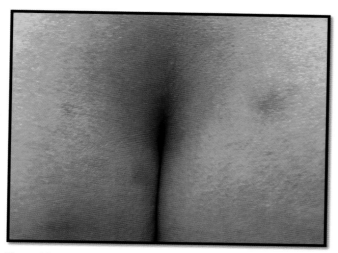

Figure 22 - HSV2. Subtle right and left buttock darkened scars from repeated past HSV2 outbreaks

2. Laboratory diagnosis:

Herpes Select – the initial, inexpensive screening test for herpes antibodies.

If *negative* (not detected) - you do not have herpes (either HSV1 or HSV2).

If *positive for HSV1 antibody* but negative for HSV2 antibody you have:

Oral HSV1 disease — if you have repeat lip, nasal or facial "cold sores."

Genital HSV1 disease — if you have classic repeated genital blister outbreaks.

Oral or genital HSV1 infection (no disease) - more likely silent oral if you have never had any suspicious skin symptoms in any location.

If *positive for HSV2 antibody at a low value* (<3.5), further confirmatory testing with HSV Western blot (a more expensive, confirmatory test that takes several weeks to return) is needed.

If *HSV2 negative by Western blot*—you do not have HSV2.

If *HSV2 positive by Western blot*—you have HSV2 infection.

If positive for HSV2 antibody at a very high value (>3.5) — you have genital HSV2 infection. HSV2 infection almost never presents orally, i.e. as cold sores.

Neither Doctor H or K know physicians who "routinely" screen their patients for genital herpes. If your doctor says you are getting a "complete STD checkup," still ask if that includes accurate herpes (and trichomonas and mycoplasma) testing. And remember, positive HSV2 blood tests need to be confirmed (with a Western blot test). Just like HIV testing, no one single test is accurate enough.

Are *Bachelor* TV contestants being unjustly discriminated when rejected based on "positive" HSV2 results?

Perhaps.

First off, the time period available to medically screen out-of-town reality show applicants is typically extremely short. Did the *Bachelor* show always run the weeks-to-return additional HSV2 confirmatory test?

Second, depending on ethnicity, individuals 20 to 40 years old (the *Bachelor* show contestant age range) have nearly a 50 percent chance of having HSV1 — HSV1 is just as likely as HSV2 to be responsible for new genital herpes infections. So, kicking off HSV2-infected, but not HSV1-infected individuals, is discriminatory — and bad medicine.

Third, the spread of HPV is potentially far more worrisome than herpes. Are contestants screened and then booted off if found positive for high-risk HPV strains? Are all potential contestants vaccinated against HPV?

ABC's the *Bachelor* is a relationship show and should take a leading role in destigmatizing STDs — especially herpes — and ending unwarranted dating hysteria. Instead, they've apparently chosen to go in the exact opposite direction.

Genital Herpes: How do you get it?

It's possible to get genital herpes merely by rubbing your skin in the "boxer shorts" regions — or having oral contact — with the "boxer shorts" skin of someone actively shedding herpes virus. Fortunately, herpes virus is not particularly contagious (see below: Infectivity - What are my chances of catching HSV?).

The herpes source typically has no herpes rash. In fact, 70 percent of new herpes cases are spread from individuals total unaware of their herpes status without any symptoms whatsoever (herpes infection, not disease). The remainder of new herpes cases are from persons aware of their herpes infection status, but who still believe they're not infectious in between — or immediately preceding — visible outbreaks.

When herpes viruses "shed," they can pass through intact skin but penetrate genital mucous membranes most readily, therefore oral, vaginal or anal sexual intercourse are riskier than lying nude and rubbing external body parts together. It also explains why twice as many females as males have genital herpes. The female genitalia — labia and vagina — have much larger and more exposed mucous membranes than the male penis. Similarly, MSM have higher rates of HSV2 and adult acquired HSV1 presumed due to receptive anal intercourse (and more exposure to bowel mucous membranes during anal intercourse).

Rarely, herpes can be passed to the hand or fingers with touching (or finger sucking), I have seen a total of two such cases, so it's rare. Fingers used to be a common location for oral herpes spread when dentists or nurses in the nursery did not wear gloves, a lesion known as herpetic whitlow.

And don't forget herpes gladiatorum. I can't. When I was a college wrestler we got our noses rubbed into the mat every day and once a year one of my colleagues picked up a new case of facial herpes from an infectious teammate unaware he was actively shedding. In an unscientific attempt to ward it off, my teammates and I would smear betadine (an orange OTC antiseptic) all over our faces. I'm not sure if it had any effect on HSV transmission, but the crazy tint looked mean as hell and we managed to place second in the NCAA championships.

Infectivity - What are my chances of catching HSV?

Fortunately, both HSV1 and HSV2 are only mildly contagious. A genital herpes-infected male will pass it a about once per 1000 episodes of vaginal sex. There are twice as many herpes infected women as men, but women pass herpes to men only half as much (once per 2000 episodes of vaginal sex). Compared with heterosexual men, MSM are two to three time as likely to have herpes (8 percent vs. 22 percent). This suggests there is a heightened transmission risk with oral and or anal sex, but more studies are needed.

About one-half of individuals with herpes have had four or fewer sex partners. On the other end of the spectrum, some people have an inborn immunity and will never succumb to the infection despite hundreds of different partners.
Herpes is most contagious during the first few hours of a classic blister attack in the initial months after getting the disease. After having herpes for a year, the amount of herpes shedding decreases then tends to stabilize. Persons with repeated painful blister outbreaks can have their herpes 'burn out' and become 'eruption free' after many years. But does silent viral shedding persist? No one knows.

In couples where one has herpes, the other doesn't, the average risk of spreading HSV2 the first year of relationship is: 3 - 4 percent for infected female with uninfected male; 5 - 10 percent for an infected male with uninfected female or uninfected male. (Remember: The more exposed mucous membranes, the more herpes susceptible).

When the herpes virus exits living skin cells, it dies within seconds. People with genital or oral herpes can use the same showers, toilets, washing machines, and swimming pools as anyone else, without the worry of lurking herpes.

Genital Herpes: Why do some get repeat outbreaks?

Repeat herpes outbreaks seem to be "triggered" by various stressors: upper respiratory tract or other infections like "the flu" or "colds" (hence the term 'cold' sores), sunlight, wind, surgery, chemotherapy or facial trauma. During a genital HSV1 or HSV2 infectious flare, viruses hibernating inside the lumbar spine suddenly go into overdrive, dispatching millions of virus particles down the nerves to, and then through, boxer-shorts-region genital skin. Most of the time, this process is symptomless, occurring through perfectly intact skin. However, in about 5 to 10 percent of the 55 million Americans with genital herpes (up to 6 million Americans), uncomfortable blisters appear a day or two after the onset of viral shedding.

Genital Herpes: Worst Case Scenarios, Including Herpes in Pregnancy

I can't say it enough.

Getting HSV infection is no big deal.

Yes, It's a nuisance. It can cause mild disease, but it's no big deal.

Getting HSV infection is no big deal.

So, what's all the stigma about? If you get herpes, what's the worst that can happen?

a) You join the 6 million (10 percent), out of the 55 million in the U.S. with genital herpes who get transient uncomfortable repeated outbreaks (mild disease). Or you join the 22 million (40 percent) with atypical, minimalistic, hard to identify herpes bouts (infection).

But again, so what? It's no big deal!

b) You are the very rare herpes infected individual (0.1 percent) who gets the uncomfortable repeat outbreaks together with low-grade headache, light hurting your eyes, stiff neck and rarely mental status changes. I've seen it in four patients in my career. While it's scary to see a young executive suddenly get all muddled up, they all get better in a few days either on their own or with antiviral medication. (serious disease but very rare).

c) You pass genital herpes to another individual (2,600,000 Americans per year) and that individual has a 10 percent chance of repeated outbreaks (mild disease) or a 0.1 percent chance of complicated outbreaks (severe disease).

d) If you are in a "herpes-only" dating site, someone with HSV1 can still transmit that infection to someone who has only HSV2, and vice versa. Having HSV1 may slightly protect you from getting HSV2. Having oral HSV1 prevents you from getting genital HSV1. But having oral HSV1 means you could give a partner genital HSV1 with oral sex.

e) You pass herpes to an immunocompromised individual at risk for more frequent and longer outbreaks.

f) You pass herpes infection to an individual at risk for HIV infection, thereby increasing the chance they get HIV two to three-fold. That translates into thousands of new HIV cases in African nations where new HIV infections are very common but is much less an issue in America.

g) The overwhelming fear? Woman diagnosed with herpes fret that an outbreak during delivery will infect their newborn. Thankfully, this disastrous complication is incredibly rare and mostly preventable. Out of about 3,800,000 American births each year, herpes is passed in only about 400-500 deliveries, and only half of those are life threatening (severe disease). Surprisingly, more than half of those infections are HSV1 (reflecting the new U.S. genital HSV1 epidemic).

Herpes testing during pregnancy

Huge debate: Should all pregnant women and their partners get blood tests for HSV1 and HSV2 antibodies?

I say yes, at least for the first child. Paradoxically, women at highest risk are those who begin their pregnancy having neither HSV1 or HSV2 (about 60 - 70 percent of moms)! Fortunately, a little education further dials down an already miniscule risk. Namely, if the woman is HSV1 negative, and her partner is oral HSV1 positive – don't receive oral sex during the second and third trimester. Or if the woman is herpes negative and the partner has HSV2 or genital HSV1 – avoid vaginal or anal sex without a condom during the second and third trimesters.

One in seven pregnant women with herpes will get a vaginal outbreak around the time of delivery that may necessitate a caesarian section. Fortunately, a highly effective prevention strategy exists: Women with genital herpes should be given anti-herpes medication the last four weeks of pregnancy. Anti-herpes medication will reduce the chance of an outbreak around the time of delivery and the need for caesarian section. Understandably, it's difficult to prospectively study the effects of drugs in newborns, but anti-herpes medication appears to be extremely safe. No significant side effects have ever been identified.

Is Herpes curable?

No.

Is Herpes treatable?

Yes. And has been for over 30 years!

There are many different doses and frequencies of herpes anti-virals, all extremely safe. In the 1990s the FDA considered allowing manufacturers to sell herpes medications over-the-counter, because side effects are practically unheard of. Infectious disease experts however successfully argued to keep antiviral medications under their control (prescription only) to help prevent drug resistance.

Common treatment protocols to treat attacks and reduce contagiousness:

1) Treatment of the first symptomatic genital HSV outbreak:
Valtrex (valacyclovir) 1000 mg twice a day x 3 days: Begin Rx immediately —even before the test results are back.

2) Treatment of repeat HSV outbreak:
Valtrex 2000 mg at first indication of attack, repeat second 2000 mg dose 12 hours later. Done. That's it.

3) Prevention of repeat symptomatic HSV outbreaks:
Valtrex 500 mg each day. This is safe to take for years at a time. Rarely, some individuals require 1000 mg per day. Prevention can also be taken episodically two to three days prior to anticipated sexual encounters.

Psych, Stigma, and Herpes: A Volatile Mix

CASE STUDY #1: A veteran rock star sheepishly walked into my medical suite with a young aspiring actress he'd recently meet. Before consummating their new relationship, fully cognizant he'd probably had a factor of a hundred more hook-ups than she, the woman demanded I run every imaginable venereal disease test. We all agreed a comprehensive STD check was prudent, but I informed the woman that by definition, comprehensive testing meant both partners test.

Fast forward: The couple sat in my inner office, apprehensively awaiting the results of a life-time of sex, drugs, and rock'n'roll with only fitful condom use. I opened up his chart first. I was thrilled to see a column of negatives (I usually learn results simultaneously with patients as the nurse files all results into charts before the face-to-face visits).

After elaborating why no HPV test had not been done (no FDA-approved test for men), I delivered the good news. He had no current STD!

The woman shot me an incredulous "no-f---ing-way" look. I handed her the rock stars' actual printout to ease her lingering doubts.

I then casually flipped open her chart. My eyes dilated. The language section of my brain froze. I handed her the lab printout, faked nonchalance but I knew she was not going to be OK with the results!

"The tests show you have both chlamydia and herpes simplex type 2 infections," I said.

There was a several beat pause.

Then, screaming at the top of her lungs, she leapt on her feet and angrily pointed a finger in the startled rocker's face. "This is a set-up!" she exploded. "You paid him to do this!"

**Moral: When it comes to STDs, you can't
always judge a book by its cover.**

CASE STUDY #2: A conservative 72-year-old man came alone to my medical suite. He matter-of-factly related that his new 55-year-old girlfriend was experiencing a vague vaginal itch for the last 3-4 days and insisted he take a thorough STD panel. She was worried about the cause as she had just resumed sexual relations with my patient after a prolonged abstinence. I agreed, but as always, I suggested he bring her in so that both sides could be tested.

They returned together, hand-in-hand, to hear his results. I sat down opposite them in my office and pulled open his chart.

"The tests show you have no Hepatitis B or C, no mycoplasma, chlamydia, gonorrhea, trichomoniasis, syphilis, or HIV. But despite your never having had symptoms or rash," I informed him, "you did test antibody-positive for Herpes Simplex Virus 2."

His face dropped, the color drained. They stopped hand-holding. The girlfriend burst into tears.

"Don't worry," I comforted her. "You've only been together for a few months. Your vaginal symptoms are not typical of herpes. Worse, worse case, the chance you've caught herpes from this relationship is less than 2 or 3 percent! And now if desired, we can start prevention to way lower future risk!"

The tearing now turned to hysterical sobbing.

"What's going through your head? What's so horrible?" I asked. In my mind I was thinking there was no chance she would ever be pregnant, so there would be no "fetus" at risk – there was no real worse case!

"Is it curable?" She sniffled.

"No," I shook my head, "but we have anti-viral drug treatment options."

"If I have it, if I were to have a new boyfriend in the future, would I have to tell him?"

"Yes, but you're talking about a mostly symptomless, treatable benign disorder. It's completely manageable!" I responded reassuringly.

The woman now wept uncontrollably again. "My life is over!"

Moral: Never underestimate HSV2 stigma and fear.

STUDY CASE #3: A patient in his early 20s presented with a painful penile rash with multiple grouped lesions. His self-diagnosis: spider bites.

After I examined him, I told him his rash was most consistent with genital herpes.

"I don't date women with herpes!" he dismissively replied. "I've been monogamous with my current girlfriend for over a year and it's impossible she gave me anything – after we started hooking up, I paid for her to have full STD testing! She was totally clear!"

He waited in my waiting room while, after getting each of the couple's consent, I requested a copy of her "Negative-for-everything STD check." I fully expected these tests to not include HSV testing — like the vast majority of outside doctor's STD checks I review. But to my surprise, HSV testing had been done. It just hadn't been properly interpreted!

Long story short: The girlfriend's lab was positive for HSV1 and negative for HSV2. She had never had an outbreak anywhere but was told, "It's oral cold sores. You have the "good" herpes."

His tests eventually revealed positive HSV1, negative HSV2, as well. So, he had gotten new symptomatic genital herpes from his girlfriend via either oral (if she silently shed HSV1 orally) or genitally (if she silently shed HSV1 genitally).

Alternatively, he could have been the source: He could have been infected with asymptomatic HSV1 all along and silently spread it to his girlfriend earlier in their relationship. Then, as can occasionally happen, some flu bug or stressor caused his asymptomatic HSV1 (infection) to morph into symptomatic genital HSV1 (disease).

Lastly, they both could have been infected long before the start of the relationship.

Moral: Patients (and doctors) routinely shrug off the "good" oral HSV1 as no big deal but gnash their teeth and scream in anguish at the thought that, God forbid, they get diagnosed with the "bad" genital HSV2. This is illogical.

Genital HSV1 and HSV2 are very very similar!

Genital HSV1 and HSV2 are very very similar

When symptomatic, genital HSV1 presents with small clusters of genital blisters, indistinguishable from HSV2 (Figures 16 and 19). Both outbreaks look exactly the same. Both outbreaks shed virus when lesions are present. Both outbreaks can shed virus silently about 3 days a month (when no lesions can be seen). In terms of the very rare chance of spread during childbirth, resulting in severe infection of the newborn, HSV1 is equal if not more of a threat than HSV2 because while HSV2 sheds more often, genital HSV1 infection is far more common.

OK, there are differences: HSV1 infection is more common than HSV2 infection – 48 percent compared to 12 percent in 15 to 49-year-old Americans. Also, compared to HSV2, genital HSV1 has fewer, milder repeat outbreaks and shedding seems to become much less common after the first year of infection.

The Surprising New STD Epidemic: Genital HSV1

It's headline news: In the U.S., *more than half of new genital herpes attacks are due to HSV1!* In one recent University study, fully 78 percent of new genital herpes was HSV1. Two recent trends are behind this startling fact.

First, only half as many American kids are getting old fashioned oral HSV1 compared to just 20 years ago. Despite nearly 80 percent plus of parents and grandparents being HSV1 positive, they are now exercising considerably more caution when kissing newborn children and grandchildren, and as a result, now only a quarter of U.S. school children get HSV1. This is in stark contrast to low income countries where essentially all children still get HSV1 (i.e. 95 percent of African children get HSV1). So, for the first time, a large percentage of American school children are susceptible if exposed to HSV1 later in life.

Second, current generations have embraced the Bill Clinton oral-pleasuring-is-not-sex view. Over the last few decades, the frequency of oral sex has increased *three-fold*. Consequently — no surprise — HSV1 from silent oral HSV1 infections is rapidly spreading via more frequent oral sex to the genitalia of susceptible HSV-negative individuals.

The face of herpes has irrevocably changed:
The HSV1 strain is not exactly "good," on the other
hand, the HSV2 strain is really not so "bad."

Herpes prevention

We are still awaiting an effective herpes vaccine. Such a breakthrough would instantly end the herpes stigma – infected persons would merely make sure their partners got the vaccine. Children could be vaccinated before they become sexually active. No one would have to think much about it after that.

Currently, those with oral HSV1 infection have a "vaccine-like" near total protection against genital HSV1. Additionally, it appears women with oral HSV1 have a three-fold lower risk of contracting HSV2 infection.

Awareness is (partial) prevention.

Studies show that when an individual is made aware of their minimal or asymptomatic genital herpes, their chance of transmitting it to a partner decreases by 50 percent. Knowledge alone reduces the spread of infection!

Three-quarters of the new herpes cases are spread by people unaware of their disease status. Based on medical studies of representative samples of the American population, as many as 50 million Americans have never noted a herpetic genital outbreak and are unaware they have genital herpes infection. It would be nice to let those folks live in ignorant bliss, but they spread three-quarters of the new cases. They need to know their status if we ever hope to control the spread of infection without a vaccine. Oddly enough, many experts (including the Centers for Disease Control) still do not include herpes testing in their "comprehensive" STD checks and discourage testing in persons at risk because of the potential "emotional harm" of incorrect diagnoses by out-of-touch doctors ordering inaccurate tests.

WHAT? Extremely accurate tests are available! We're not going to test because a large percentage of doctors can't gasp the proper testing paradigm? Are you kidding me? Prompt awareness of herpes and early initiation of education should be the goal for both patients and doctors.

Why do doctors omit HSV testing from "comprehensive" STD screens?

1. Doctors are skittish about talking to patients about sex.
2. Doctors have no time to handle the inevitable newly-diagnosed-herpes-freak-outs. Why not let the millions with silent herpes infections live in ignorant bliss? Some doctors "sidestep" herpes stigma by telling patients with obvious genital herpes outbreaks they have shingles, a similarly appearing viral infection that, also, like both strains of herpes simplex responds to valtrex (valacyclovir). Our sworn oath after all, is *primum non nocere*. Above all, do no harm.
3. No doctor wants the nightmare of giving a patient a false-positive (wrong) result. Neophyte doctors often misinterpret cheaper herpes screening tests as positive for HSV2 antibody when more accurate tests show negative for HSV2 antibody. Confirmation of a positive first test HSV2 antibody test is critical.

4. No doctor wants to give a patient a false-negative (wrong) result – you cannot tell a patient he doesn't have genital herpes based on a negative HSV2 antibody test. The patient may in fact have genital HSV1 infection. There's an accurate blood test for HSV1 antibody, but a positive HSV1 antibody test can indicate either oral or genital HSV1 infection. Because HSV1 can infect either the oral or genital skin, a positive HSV1 antibody blood test cannot determine the site of infection.
5. Herpes has no compelling long-term bodily harm.
6. Herpes has no compelling individual treatment. There is no herpes vaccine, despite repeated promises over the last 40 years. Antiviral drugs, condoms, telling the partner of one's HSV diagnosis and education as to the appearance of atypical HSV outbreaks are each individually only partially effective. As a group, however, they are probably extremely effective, as evidenced by the surprising 33 percent drop in herpes cases in the U.S. over the last 15 years.
7. Misinterpreted herpes tests may lead to unnecessary caesarean sections if doctors don't know the exact transmission risks and do not know about the safety and benefits of anti-herpes medication in the third trimester of pregnancy.
8. Many doctors blindly follow CDC recommendations which dissuade (for all the wrong reasons!) doctors from screening for new HSV infections.

Treatment is (partial) prevention

Anti-herpes drugs — acyclovir, valacyclovir (Valtrex) or famciclovir (Famvir) — partially suppress both symptomatic outbreaks and asymptomatic herpes shedding. They're less successful at suppressing elevated viral loads at the start of visible herpes attacks. Some get total protection, while others get less or no benefit. Overall, daily anti-herpes drug use lowers the chance of herpes transmission by 50 percent.

Anti-herpes medications are very safe. The medications have no effect on human cells and at usual doses only very rarely have side effects (i.e., headache).

Herpes pre-exposure prophylaxis (PrEP)?

Using anti-herpes drugs (acyclovir, valacyclovir or famciclovir) is beneficial if taken in anticipation of outbreak triggers like sun exposure, surgery, general infections, severe stress or chemotherapy.

Should a herpes-free person pop a 1000 mg valacyclovir before sex with someone who has herpes? There are no studies evaluating this preventative approach, but it could work. The recent wildly successful use of Truvada and doxycycline before sex (pre-exposure prophylaxis) to prevent HIV, syphilis and chlamydia in at risk individuals suggests that if valacyclovir worked, people would take it. A study needs to be done.

I think herpes pre-exposure prophylaxis (PrEP) is a reasonable option.

I personally don't think herpes is a big deal, but if you do, and you're certain you do not already have herpes, I suggest an unproven but scientifically plausible prevention: Take 1000 mg valacyclovir pill one to three hours before intercourse if you know or suspect your partner has herpes. FYI: Valacyclovir costs up to $2 per pill and medical insurance will not cover a drug such as this used in a non-FDA approved manner.

Dr. K disagrees with me. He thinks a study should be done — and if it shows a benefit — only then would he recommend herpes PrEP.

Protection is (partial) prevention

The regular use of condoms lowers the risk of herpes transmission by 50 percent. Condoms work better in preventing male-to-female compared to female-to-male transmission of HSV (remember females have more exposed mucous membranes than men).

As mentioned before, condoms slip or fall off or are misused 20 - 30 percent of the time in real-world usage. Equally pertinent, genital herpes can shed anywhere in the "boxer short" region, and condoms only cover a portion of the shaft of the penis.

Talking is (partial) prevention

Roughly 6 million Americans have experienced the classic uncomfortable blistering herpes genital rash. Most of them "know" they have herpes. Of this group, a clear majority (80 percent) do not disclose their status to new partners. Roughly 50 million Americans have asymptomatic genital herpes infection. Very few of them "know" they have herpes, so only a few of these individuals are in a position to disclose their infection.

No one knows exactly what percent of couples break up due to an honest disclosure of genital herpes. In couples that stay together, studies show that disclosing the genital herpes diagnosis to your partner lowers the risk of transmission by 50 percent. Somehow, someway, these couples manage to avoid contact more often during detectable flares or use other preventative measure more effectively.

DOCTORS H AND K RECOMMEND:
Always fully disclose your herpes status to your partner(s). If a relationship cannot weather the herpes storm, it's not likely to endure the far bigger storms of finances or child raising.

Be aware that many states have counterproductive laws that "criminalize" herpes. (See STDs and the Law.)

Full court genital herpes prevention: *if you don't have it*

1. Test yourself if you are:
   a. Beginning a new sexual relationship.
   b. Experiencing unexplained genital skin sensitivity, rash or urinary discomfort.
   c. Pregnant.
      i. If positive (initial screening HSV2 "positives" may need to be confirmed by additional tests), consider antiviral medication to reduce the frequency of viral shedding during labor, thereby reducing the need for cesarean delivery.
      ii. If testing is negative (no antibodies detected), discuss the need for male partner testing to reduce the chance of getting either genital HSV1 or HSV2 late in the pregnancy thereby increasing the risk of transmission to the newborn during vaginal delivery.
   d. High risk for sexually acquiring HSV1 or HSV2 infections.
      i. Men who have sex with men.
      ii. Sex workers.
      iii. Men who employ sex workers.
      iv. IV drug users.
      v. Those with 10 - 20 or more lifetime sex partners.
2. Test your partners. Remember it takes 4 weeks for the usual herpes tests to turn positive. If a partner is positive, suggest they:

a. take antiviral medication.
b. use condoms.
c. learn about atypical HSV presentations.
d. avoid sex during outbreaks.

3. Check out your doctors, many don't know how to properly test! Make sure they use a two-step type-specific testing process with confirmation, account for the window period and consider increasingly common genital HSV1 infections.
4. Use condoms (50 percent reduced risk).
5. Ask. However, only 10 to 20 percent of herpes patients are aware and only about 20 percent of them will be truthful.
6. Examine. 5 - 10 percent have possible telltale scars from the episodic HSV outbreaks.
7. Avoid pubic grooming. If you must go hairless, groom at least two days prior to sexual contact.
8. Educate. Learn how oral, vaginal, and rectal sex and skin-to-skin contact (anywhere in "boxer shorts" region) might spread herpes.
9. *Unproven but scientifically plausible approaches:*
   a. Pre-exposure prophylaxis (HSV1/HSV2 "PrEP") with valacyclovir or acyclovir before sex.
   b. Maintain health with regular exercise, well balanced diet, and adequate sleep for optimization of your immune system.

Full court herpes prevention: if know you have genital herpes

1. Tell your partner. Just this disclosure alone markedly lowers your chance of passing the virus to your partner (50 percent reduced risk).
2. Take antiviral medication daily (50 percent reduced risk).
3. Educate. Find out if you're having classic "mini" outbreaks and abstain from sex during these heightened obvious or minimally symptomatic' infectious flares.
4. Avoid pubic grooming. If you must go hairless, groom at least two to three days prior to sexual contact.
5. Test new partners for HSV; if positive, anti-herpes preventative measures may not be necessary. In other words, if both partners have HSV1 or both have HSV2, no further spread can occur. You cannot infect a partner if they are positive with the same HSV strain as you.
6. Know how herpes spreads: oral sex, vaginal intercourse, rectal intercourse, and skin-to-skin contact (anywhere in "boxer shorts" region).
7. *Unproven but scientifically plausible approaches:*
   a. Have potential partners take anti-herpes medication before sex (HSV PrEP).
   b. Shingles vaccine (one small study showed decreased symptomatic outbreaks).

c. Maintain healthy immune system with regular exercise, well balanced diet, and adequate sleep as a means of optimizing your immune system.

Alternate, ethically dicey approach for those willing to stretch the truth - as recommended grudgingly by several pragmatic gynecologists I know – but not endorsed by Doctors H or K!

It's true, some men will drop a woman (and vice-a-versa) like a hot potato if they admit up front they have genital herpes. Because of this irrational stigma, I am aware of several excellent doctors in our community who advise their patients not to tell partners unless directly asked (most partners don't ask) all the while using condoms and taking anti-herpes meds and avoiding encounters if any symptoms exist.

After a couple of sexual encounters during which there is a less than a one-in-a-thousand chance of spreading the herpes, tell your partner you might have herpes. This is true because in the past some out of touch doctors have relied on inaccurate testing and you are on a daily protective anti-viral medication, which in some cases may be fully protective.

However, honesty from the start is usually better in the end. Also, many states still have laws that make this "reasonable" approach illegal.

Part III - BACTERIAL STDs — All Curable with Antibiotics (For Now!)

CHAPTER 12
Syphilis: The Great Imitator

"The physician who knows syphilis knows medicine." — *Sir William Osler*

Syphilis is inextricably intertwined with American history.

When Christopher Columbus and his sailors discovered the New World in 1492, they and the European explorers that followed in quick succession brought along a Pandora's box of diseases: bubonic plague, cholera, diphtheria, malaria, scarlet fever, smallpox, gonorrhea, and tuberculosis. Epidemics of these diseases over the ensuing years decimated much of the native Indian population.

Columbus and his men, in return, were exposed to a disease found only in certain Western Hemisphere tribes: syphilis. In the years after Columbus's return to Spain, syphilis spread like a dry season wildfire, devastating a susceptible European population. At its zenith, one in five Europeans suffered from this crippling bacterial disease with one notable complication even worse than death — syphilis dementia. Chris Columbus, Henry VIII, Bram Stoker, Vincent van Gogh, Ivan the Terrible, Al Capone, Vladimir Lenin, and Hitler appear to all have been afflicted with this personality altering end stage complication characterized by delusions of grandeur, loss of inhibitions, pathological lying and loss of cognitive function. (Do we test our current day politicians — on both sides of the aisle - for syphilis during their executive physicals?)

Syphilis infected a huge number of Americans before WWII — up to 10 percent based on autopsy studies. Then, as blood tests and antibiotics became available in the 1950s, syphilis was nearly eliminated, leading optimists to predict disease eradication was imminent.

I spent half my medical school years studying syphilis. Yes, the inordinate study hours were partly because STDs fascinated me, but also because these resilient bacteria hold a sacred place in medical education. Syphilis is reverently called "the great imposter" and seemingly 25 percent of exam questions were based on syphilis trivia. The corkscrew bacterium infiltrates every single body organ, ergo it may mimic any disease in the books, whether heart, brain, bone or intestine. When I was on ward rounds as a medical student and had no idea what was going on, I'd buy time by saying "could be atypical syphilis" for guaranteed brownie points while struggling to formulate my real answer.

Understandably, I graduated primed to diagnose and treat every tricky syphilitic iteration. Yet, despite looking literally under every rock for this history changing STD, as a private doctor in Beverly Hills, with over 200,000 patient encounters, I've diagnosed fewer than 10 cases! None of these cases were subtle. All had obvious risk factors – either MSM with hundreds of encounters or several pro athletes spending a chunk of their game checks at "Nude, Nude, Nude," a strip joint down the street from LAX.

My "expertise" did come in handy a decade ago when a syphilis blood test was a California marriage license requirement (now only in Mississippi). Every few months I'd get a dire emergency call – a bride or groom-to-be in meltdown mode after being told they had syphilis! Fortunately, I could be the hero by explaining how incredibly rare syphilis was and why this initial screening test was almost certainly a *false positive*. In several days when the more accurate confirmatory test returned — proving they did not really have syphilis — I had a friend for life.

But now this incredibly infectious corkscrew syphilis bacterium is making an improbable comeback. Syphilis rates in the U.S., have increased 76 percent over the last 4 years! Syphilis rates are now are three times higher than just a decade ago. World-wide, 8 million new cases occur yearly just in South East Asia and Sub-Saharan Africa.

In total, how many Americans are infected with syphilis?

120,000.

How many Americans get new infections each year?

88,000 (2016) (this is up 18 percent from 2015). This number is higher than the official CDC tally as some cases are kept "secret" and not reported and others are never properly diagnosed.

Only one-third were caught in the earliest stage, eliminating any chance of permanent complications. MSM and bisexual men accounted for 70 percent of all new cases, although MSM number less than 10 percent of all sexually active men.

There were about 628 new congenital cases in 2016 — syphilis passed from pregnant women to their babies — essentially double the number compared to 2012 (334 cases).

How do you get syphilis?

The syphilis bacterium easily passes through intact mucous membrane or abraded (i.e. shaved) skin. You get syphilis via oral, vaginal and or anal sexual contact with infectious skin lesions. Because it is passed skin to skin, condoms are only partially effective (50 percent). It can be passed by kissing when a tongue or mouth syphilitic sore is present. A pregnant woman can pass the syphilis bacterium via blood through the placenta to the developing fetus. Rarely, syphilis has been passed via blood transfusions. The syphilis bacterium is unable to survive outside the body. It does not live on toilet seats or gym equipment.

What are the first warning signs of syphilis?

A painless, firm half-inch growth appears on the penis, outer labia, perianal region, lip, tongue or inside the mouth or throat at the site of initial sexual contact.

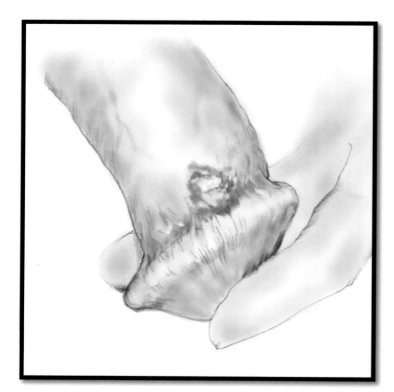

Figure 23 - Syphilis. A painless distal penile chancer, appearing just under the glans

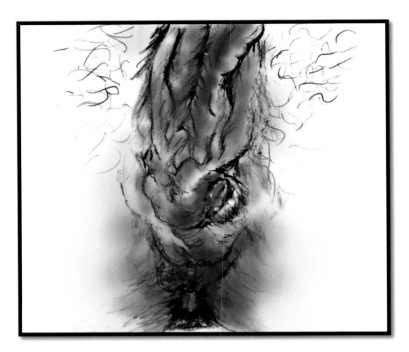

Figure 24 - Syphilis. An indurated, painless left labial chancer

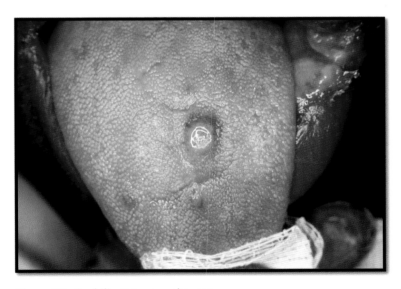

Figure 25 - Syphilis. A tongue chancer

After about a week, the raised lesion ulcerates with the open center surrounded by slightly raised borders. Painless lymph nodes may also appear, especially if the exposed sore gets secondarily infected. The primary syphilitic lesion may not be apparent in women (inner vagina or cervix) or in MSM (inner rectum).

What is the usual course of syphilis if you don't treat?

Primary stage: Syphilis bacteria penetrate intact mucous membranes or skin, especially damaged (i.e. shaved) genital skin. Within days, the immune system kicks in, attempting to keep the infection local. However, within a few weeks, the bacteria win the battle. Shortly thereafter, infectious bacteria begin to emerge through superficial syphilitic sores (chancers).

The time from sexual contact to the development of an initial painless sore averages three weeks, but the sore can show up as early as 10 days or as late as 3 months. The syphilitic "chancers" I've seen were dime sized open sores with heaped-up edges, nothing like the smaller groups of uncomfortable shallow herpes ulcers that I see practically daily. The chancer disappears in three to six weeks even if no antibiotics are given. However, the infection persists and soon progresses to the secondary stage.

Secondary stage: One to three months after the primary sore, the syphilis bacteria multiply throughout the body and reemerge as skin rashes and/or sores in the mouth, vagina, or anus along with fever, swollen lymph nodes, and muscle and joint aches. The rash is measles-like, involves the palms and the soles, but occasionally exhibits scaly features on par with psoriasis. Patchy scalp and beard hair loss can occur as well. About 2 - 5 percent of the time additional symptoms may occur such as blurred vision, hearing loss or ringing in the ears or headaches. Those symptoms can point to early syphilis of the brain, so in high risk settings, it's important not to blow off these complaints! A timely diagnosis can avert the very real chance of neurological damage.

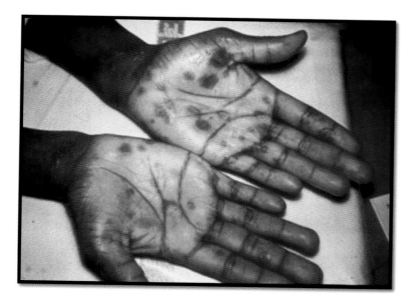

Figure 26 - Syphilis. Secondary stage syphilis with classic involvement of the palms and soles

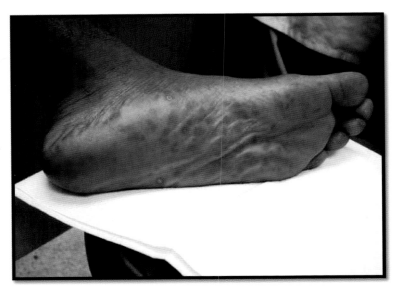

Figure 27 - Syphilis. Secondary stage syphilis with classic involvement of the palms and soles

Like primary syphilis, the myriad symptoms of secondary syphilis disappear spontaneously. However, without treatment, 25 percent of the time, syphilis progresses to the dreaded "third stage."

Third stage: Basically, the body gives us two swings in the early innings of the syphilis game. After that, 75 percent luck out and their syphilis spontaneously goes away. But for the other 25 percent, it's Katie Bar the Door! They progress over a decade or more to catastrophic eye, heart, blood vessel, or brain and spinal cord damage. The frontpage disaster is progressive dementia. It begins subtly with irritability, memory lapses, faulty speech, or personality changes. Congenital syphilis: Syphilis bacteria readily cross the placental barrier, infect the fetus, and often cause spontaneous abortion or still births. If the infected baby lives, abnormalities of the teeth, bones and later progressive brain damage are to be expected.

How is syphilis diagnosed?

Syphilis is diagnosed via blood tests but you have to suspect it and *request* testing. Syphilis is the great imposter: It can mimic hundreds of different diseases. Even though it's relatively rare, stay on guard.

Get a test if you have unexplained open genital sores, vaginal or rectal bleeding, swollen groin lymph nodes, fever, aches, severe headaches, weird brain problems, or an unexplained measles-like rash — especially if it involves the palms and soles!

Get a test if you are pregnant.

Get a screening test every three months regardless of symptoms if you are:
1. Sexually active non-monogamous MSM
2. HIV-infected and sexually active
3. Taking PrEP for HIV prevention
4. Heterosexual with a recent STD or with new or multiple partners (an annual blood test recommended here)

What are the syphilis blood tests?

Screening tests: VDRL or RPR blood tests can be done quickly and inexpensively. They turn positive approximately 21 days (10 - 90 days) after exposure. About 2 percent of the time a positive test is misleading: The person does not have syphilis (a false positive). That is the reason I had so many "pre-wedding"-false-alarm-syphilis-emergencies. False positives are especially common in the presence of Lyme disease (which just so happens to be a relative of syphilis), mononucleosis, lupus or other autoimmune diseases.

Confirmation tests: If the screening VDRL or RPR test is positive, it must be confirmed with tests for treponemal antibodies specific for syphilis (FTA-Ab, TP-EIA or TPPA). Those antibodies appear very early in the disease (7 - 10 days) and remain detectable for life, even after successful treatment. A negative treponemal antibody test excludes syphilis infection.

Is syphilis curable?

Yes. In the early stages, it's 100 percent curable.

For pregnant women, penicillin treatment early in pregnancy is 95 percent effective in preventing mother-to-child transmission. Unless the mom is allergic, penicillin is extremely safe to both mother and child.

Still, if you are cured of syphilis that doesn't mean you can't get re-infected later in life. In fact, bacterial STDs — like gonorrhea, chlamydia, mycoplasma and syphilis — are all curable but in all instances, re-exposure can cause re-infection. It seems unfair. Isn't our immune response supposed to prevent repeat infections? It turns out these STD bacteria have evolved a clever mechanism to evade the body's powerful antibodies designated to fatally puncture the bacteria's thick cell wall. These bacteria defend themselves by continually changing the markers on the outside of their thick cell wall.

Viruses cannot do this as readily — viruses are much smaller and simpler than bacteria — small changes in the DNA of the virus make it non-viable. Once our immune system recognizes and eliminates a viral infection, like hepatitis A or measles, we get life-long protection.

Is syphilis treatable?

Yes. The ideal treatment though depends on how early syphilis is discovered. The longer syphilis has percolated in the body, the greater the dose and duration of the penicillin needed to effect a cure.

Primary or secondary syphilis or syphilis of less than one-year duration:

Benzathine penicillin G 2.4 million units intramuscularly, one dose.

Ouch. Treated people need to abstain from sexual contact for 7 days.

Syphilis of unknown duration with absolutely no signs or symptoms:

Benzathine penicillin G 7.2 million units total, given as 2.4 million units intramuscularly per week, three weeks in a row.

Ouch. Ouch. Ouch. Treated people need to abstain from sexual contact for 21 days.

Third stage disease - Any evidence of eye, heart, or brain involvement:

Crystalline penicillin G 18 - 24 million units IV/day for 14 days followed by 1-3 shots as above.

Ouch or Ouch, ouch, ouch. Treatment will prevent disease progression but may not reverse the damage already done.

What are my chances of catching syphilis?

Syphilis is extremely infectious. It's four hundred-fold more infectious than HIV via vaginal sex. If you have sex just once with someone with syphilis, you have a 30 percent chance of getting it. After 10 exposures to someone with infectious syphilis, there is a 97 percent chance syphilis was transmitted.

Syphilis – HIV connection

Syphilis increases odds both of getting HIV or transmitting HIV up to five-fold. More than 50 percent of MSM in the U.S. diagnosed with syphilis also have HIV. Untreated HIV-infected individuals can have more rapid progression to brain damaging syphilis leading to blindness or deafness. Syphilis also increases the HIV viral load (making someone more infectious for HIV) and decreases the

CD4 T cell count (making someone more immunosuppressed and hastening the progression of untreated HIV).

Syphilis prevention

Awareness is prevention
Centuries before curative antibiotics, yesteryear's brothels would employ a "cock" lady to examine patrons and refuse entry to anyone with suspicious skin lesions. Without question, every adolescent and young adult should be educated today on the visual presentation of syphilis as well as STDs in general.

However, knowing now that most STDs have no symptoms at all, it's apparent the well intentioned "cock lady's" approach was flawed. Still, knowing what STDs can look like is at times extremely useful and an important way to be empowered and to protect yourself and others by getting tested and treated early.

Once a diagnosis is made, persons with syphilis must notify all recent sex partners (the lab that runs the test must also report all positive tests to county health officials). Given syphilis's high infectivity, it makes emotional and economic sense to treat all contacts immediately, even before their test results are available. Remember, syphilis tests are not reliable until at least a full 3 - 12 weeks after contact.

Treatment is prevention
Complying with the full treatment course and waiting for all syphilis lesions to disappear prevents the possibility of future syphilis transmission.

Protection is prevention
Never "pubic groom" within two days of planned romantic liaison. Damaged skin can facilitate the transmission of the syphilis bacterium, which readily passes through skin. Condoms are only 50 percent effective at prevention. Syphilis can be transferred through genital skin not covered by a condom and via oral lesions.

Far and away the most surreal STD case I've ever seen was a gentleman who threw a New Year's Eve party and kissed all the guests as they arrived. Days later, an oral syphilitic ulcer was discovered. He had to call each and every holiday guest and have them go for a benzathine penicillin shot!

Prophylaxis is prevention
Recent studies in gay populations at high risk for syphilis — for instance those taking HIV PrEP and not using condoms — can markedly lower their chance of catching syphilis (and chlamydia) when they take 100 mg of doxycycline daily or 200 mg of doxycycline one time before or immediately after every dicey (i.e. no condom, no recent STD testing by partner) hook-up.

This is no longer idle speculation given the dramatic recent surge in bacterial STDs (syphilis, chlamydia, and gonorrhea) seemingly associated with the rise of online dating apps facilitating casual one time meet-ups together with less condom use (a recent teen survey noted use of condoms with last sexual contact had dropped from 60 percent to 53 percent over the last 10 years).

High-risk behaviors (social media arranged anonymous sex, condom-less sex, multiple partners, sex under the influence of drugs and alcohol, and the under 25 age group where anonymous sexual hook-ups are more socially acceptable) clearly are linked to recent surging STD infection rates.

County health departments, already stretched thinly between increasing numbers of STDs, slashed budgets and reduced STD services, are now facing a larger challenge: tracking down online dating partners with no known last name or contact information. It doesn't help that in some of the hardest hit states — are you listening Utah? — only abstinence is taught in school sex-ed classes.

CHAPTER 13
Open Genital Sores: Other Bacterial STD Causes

You see red bumps. Within days they morph into open genital sores. You probably have herpes.

Less likely, the open genital sores are weird bug bites or a dermatologic condition like shingles, bullous pemphigus or lichen planus. Syphilis is unlikely — but you absolutely can't afford to miss this possibility.

For completeness, I'm mentioning three rare (in the U.S.) bacterial STDs — Chancroid, Granuloma Inguinale, and Lymphogranuloma Venereum (LGV) — that cause genital ulcers.

If your genital sores are unresponsive or atypical, especially if you've been traveling outside the U.S. or you are a male who has had sex with a male (MSM), spend a moment studying the following:

Chancroid is caused by a bacterium transmitted sexually from the open sores of an infected person (similar to syphilis). Typically, half of those infected develop an asymptomatic carrier state, half have an irritating red dot suddenly pop up in the genitalia or anus five to seven days after exposure. Within a matter of hours, the bump morphs into a painful soft open sore (as differentiated from the painless, hard syphilis sore) with nearby painfully enlarged lymph nodes. Obviously, in women, skin findings are harder to appreciate and symptoms are tricky as well, the vaginal lesions presenting as pain on urination or pain with intercourse.

There are just a handful of U.S. chancroid cases reported yearly, but it remains in low income countries, especially among urban sex workers. Currently, tests are limited to large laboratories or research centers, so the diagnosis is old school: a history of sexual exposure, travel, and painful genital sore(s) and lymph nodes, with negative syphilis tests.

Untreated, lymph nodes scar or occasionally rupture before the entire infection resolves spontaneously in two to three months. But this disease can still kill. Open ulcers jack HIV transmission by as much as 300 percent.

Chancroid is easily treatable:

Azithromycin 1 gram by mouth one time

As always, contact all partners within the prior 60 days.

Granuloma Inguinale is caused by a mildly contagious bacterium, seen more typically in steady rather than one-night stand partners. After a long, up to ten-week incubation, a distinctive, sharply demarcated ulcer — painless, firm, beefy red and prone to ooze blood — gradually forms. In women, internal vaginal lesions have been reported to cause vaginal or rectal bleeding. Self-touching can spread the rash, especially to the peri-rectal perineal skin. There are usually no associated swollen glands. It's unknown how many carriers exist.

Granuloma Inguinale like chancroid has no easily available blood test, so diagnosis hinges heavily on recognizing the beefy red, easily oozing genital ulcer(s).

Granuloma Inguinale is fully treatable. The antibiotics need to be continued considerably longer than for most STDs:

Doxycycline 100 mg twice a day x 3 week
or
Ciprofloxacin 750 mg twice a day x 3 week

Given the exceptionally long time between when you first got the infection and when the external infectious rash first appears, it's necessary to contact all partners within the prior 90 days.

Lymphogranuloma Venereum (LGV), a unique strain of chlamydia that can cause swollen glands and gastrointestinal infection, is another uncommon STD in the U.S. (except in the gay male community) that presents with open genital sores — or sometimes with absolutely no symptoms at all. About three days to three weeks after exposure, the symptomatic group (a third of the total group) get small herpes-like open sores on genital skin, but in contrast to herpes, these are painless. The lesions heal within days and do not scar. In MSM, the first sign may be anal pain, bloody rectal discharge and fever, symptomatically similar to inflammatory bowel disease (Crohn's disease or ulcerative colitis). One to four weeks after the ulcerative rash, tender swollen glands appear in the groin, occasionally filling-up with pus and then spontaneously draining — an "alien-like" experience with residual scarring.

Left untreated, about 5 percent may develop scarring and strictures of the penis, urethra, scrotum, rectum, and vulva. Worse case, the lymphatic drainage is obliterated and the resultant edema produces elephantiasis of the penis. (Beware what you wish for!)

I've seen a grand total of one case in my life time — but it's making a come-back among MSM in Europe and the U.S.

Diagnosis is based on transient painless genital ulcers (if present), painful genital lymph nodes, and in MSM rectal pain, discharge, and bleeding. Rectal swabs for chlamydia PCR are accurate in the latter scenario but cannot distinguish between LGV and standard type chlamydia.

Excellent treatment exists:

Doxycycline 100 mg twice/d x 3 weeks or
Azithromycin 1 gram orally each week x 3 weeks

Of course, all sexual contacts over the prior 60 days should be contacted.

Bacterial STDs with Genital and Peri-Rectal Ulcers

Disease	Ulcers	Lymph nodes	Diagnosis
Syphilis	painless	none	Two-step blood test
Chancroid (Hemophilus Ducreyi)	painful	multiple, tender	culture
Granuloma Inguinale (Klebsiella Granulomatis)	painless bleeds easily beefy red	none	culture
Lymphogranuloma Venereum (C Trachomatis)	Painless, small, herpes-like sores	Multiple, tender 0.5% - 1% MSM may have LGV rectal proctitis or colonization	DNA swab test

Table 8

CHAPTER 14
Gonorrhea – The Clap

Gonorrhea is the STD standard bearer: an incredibly deceptive, nasty and infectious pathogen that's as relevant today as it was thousands of years ago. The Bible clearly describes gonorrheal "urethral discharge" and the associated disgust, shame, and perceived uncleanliness. Flash forward to today: The biblical description pretty much still holds true! But the latest internet headlines show gonorrhea is staying very current. A brand new southeast Asian "super-strain" resistant to last-resort antibiotics was just documented in a London man after a Thailand vacation.

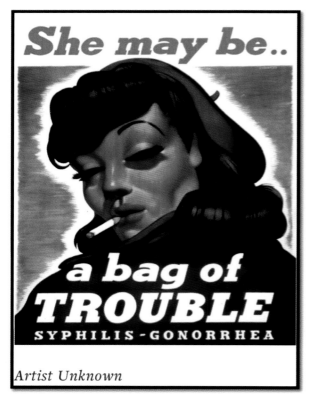

Artist Unknown

Figure 28 - The age-old belief that women are to blame for a disproportionate amount of gonorrhea is false

The "clap" moniker derives from the Le Clapier district of Paris, now the 4th arrondissement, where prostitutes were housed in the Middle Ages. Back then, and for centuries to follow, "bad" women were generally blamed as the source of this scourge.

Of course, this is preposterous. True, twice as many women as men have gonorrhea, but during vaginal sex, men are twice as infectious as woman. So, men give the same amount of gonorrhea they get.

Back in the day, the clap was bad. Imagine pus dripping non-stop out the penis, rectum, or vagina. But the remedies inserted up urethras were even worse: caustic chemicals or lubrication-free "soundings" with metal catheters of all sizes. In the mid eighteenth century, Dr. Hunter, an infamous English surgeon, tried to figure the clap out, only to show how wrong even well-intentioned science can go. He injected himself with the blood of a gonorrhea patient and got syphilis! He then proceeded to claim (*A Treatise on the Venereal Diseases*, 1786) that gonorrhea and syphilis were the same STD. (For the record, some scholars believe this woeful experiment was in fact performed on a hapless human test subject — not by Dr. Hunter on himself).

Finally, in 1879, the cause of gonorrhea was discovered – a bacteria. The bacterium was ultimately named *Neisseria gonorrhoeae* after the discoverer: Dr. Albert Neisser. Gonorrhea became just the second disease-causing bacteria isolated (Anthrax famously being the first). Still, humane and effective therapy had to wait – antibiotics were not discovered for another 50 years.

Sulfonamide drugs and penicillin became available in 1936 and 1943 respectively. Those momentous drug discoveries saved lives the instant they were released. Yet, it didn't take long before a chilling cat-and-mouse game between antibiotics and wily bacteria played out around the world. About one third of all gonorrhea strains developed resistance to sulfa by 1944. Penicillin worked well until 1976 when resistant strains originating in the Far East became common. Tetracycline resistance occurred about ten years later. *Neisseria gonorrhoeae* figured a way around ciprofloxacin by about 2007. That's when a two-drug regimen was instituted to prevent the emergence of any more resistant strains.

Guess what? In 2018 a new gonorrhea strain was identified resistant to our last-resort two-drug combination! Who knows if this strain will gain a foothold? The capability of the gonorrhea bacteria to mutate allowing the development of resistance to multiple antibiotics is one of today's most frightening world health dilemmas.

The capability of the gonorrhea bacteria to mutate allowing the development of resistance to multiple antibiotics is one of today's most frightening world health dilemmas.

How many people are currently infected with gonorrhea in the U.S.?

250,000.

The military is typically a high-risk group: 2 percent of our soldiers are currently infected.

How many get new gonorrhea infections each year?

820,000.

This represents a whopping 67 percent increase over just the last four years. Many cases are not reported to county health officials. Private patients are not thrilled having their name added to a county STD registry — even if local health officials swear this is "confidential" information.

Worldwide, there are probably around 78 million new cases per year. Scariest statistic? Gonorrhea rates among pregnant women in South Africa are 8 percent! (Yes, babies can get gonorrhea of the eyes during childbirth leading to blindness.)

How is gonorrhea acquired?

You get the clap when an infected source — vagina, penile urethra, rectum, throat, saliva or occasionally fingers — contacts a mucous membrane lining (i.e. the vagina, urethra, rectum, throat). Saliva as source of transmission may be more likely than we think. Australian studies show some men spread gonorrhea via deep kissing without any sexual contact.

You can get gonorrhea multiple times. Dr. K had one patient at the San Francisco STD Clinic who had it 36 times. Bad luck, bad genes or a really bad online dating app?

Neisseria gonorrhoeae can live outside the body for a few hours so infection from shared towels or bathroom items (especially if they remain a little moist) is reported on rare occasions.

What are the first warning signs of gonorrhea?

Two to seven days after contact, men who get symptoms initially complain of a scant penile drip which intensifies over 24 hours to an undeniable thick pus accompanied by urinary burning (Figure 28).

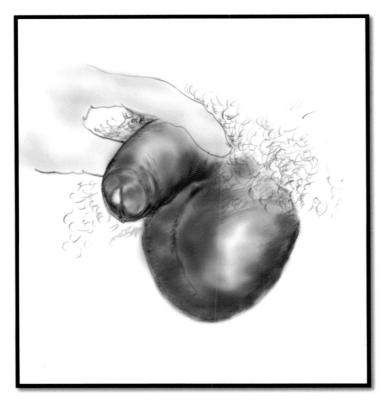

Figure 29 - Gonorrhea. Thick pus discharge (white blood cells) from the penis

Women who get symptoms may notice a thin, purulent, mildly malodorous vaginal discharge with some pain on urination. Throat and anal infections show up less dramatically, but MSM who have symptoms might complain of sore throat, rectal itchiness, scant rectal mucous discharge and the urge to defecate.

What if you don't treat?

When guys get gonorrhea, most get obvious pus dripping from the penis. Not surprisingly, they seek medical care pronto. About 25 percent get only thin, minimalistic, "chlamydia-like" discharge. They seek treatment on a less urgent basis. The minority of infected men with no discharge, no burning, no nothing, typically remain undiagnosed and untreated, unknowingly spreading gonorrhea to others.

As far as gonorrhea is concerned, women are not as fortunate as men. Only half get infection symptoms despite all having exam evidence of cervix and urethral inflammation/discharge. Gonorrhea may infect the throat or tonsils though throat pain is usually minimal. About 40 percent of woman with gonorrhea also have rectal involvement, most without admitted anal sex, presumably spread from cervical discharge. Up to 40 percent of MSM have primary rectal infection.

Sexually active with an unexplained pus-filled pink eye? Auto inoculation of *Neisseria gonorrhoeae* from the urethra to the eye is occasionally seen. Promptly seek treatment to prevent this vision altering blight.

Untreated, gonorrhea typically festers for several months at the initial contact site then four-fifths of the time burns out and spontaneously clears over six months. However, 20 percent of the time, the *Neisseria gonorrhoeae* bacterium meanders up the genital tract intent on damaging the internal reproductive organs.

Bad outcomes occur mainly in women — pelvic inflammatory disease (PID) being the all-too-common gonorrhea endgame. One episode of PID increases ectopic pregnancy ten-fold, leaves 15 percent of woman infertile and can kick off gut twisting chronic pelvic pain even when antibiotics are immediately administered.

Working ER shifts after my Cedars Sinai internship day-job, I'd run from minor dramas to full on disasters all night long, but as sleep deprived as I was, I'll never forget one patient exhibiting the textbook physical finding of PID: the *"Chandelier"* sign. (You read about disease presentations all day long in medical school, but it's still jolting when you actually experience it). At 4 a.m. a hysterical teen presented with nagging abdominal pain, claiming she couldn't sleep. I, of course, was less than sympathetic on that front. Her abdominal exam wasn't suggestive of either gall stones or appendicitis, my first two thoughts. So, I proceeded to perform a pelvic exam. As the initial step, two gloved fingers are inserted and the cervix is gently manipulated both up and down. Immediately, all hell broke loose! She let out a blood-curdling rebel yell, her body literally rising off the gurney with arms flailing upward as if to grab an imaginary ceiling light —a positive *chandelier* sign — maybe the most haunting exam-based provocative test in all of medicine.

Other Big Bang complications: *Neisseria gonorrhoeae* occasionally sneaks into the blood stream with a proclivity to settle in joints and skin. Swollen, achy, stiff joints? Sudden Achilles pain (lover's heels)? Pustular rash? Women by virtue of higher frequency of silent/symptomless gonorrhea or symptoms masked by menstruation or pregnancy are much more prone to get these complications. Orthopedic injuries have always been a special interest of mine, but when an adolescent limps into my office with no history of trauma, I don't think orthopedics — I think gonorrhea.

How is gonorrhea diagnosed?

Diagnosis used to be punitive: Even the slightest urinary burn symptom would necessitate the doctor twisting a cotton Q tip up the urethra for a culture specimen. The cultures had to be immediately run back to the lab and plated on an esoteric petri culture disc with iffy success. Now it's night and day easier — and more humane. Urine (or if indicated patient self-collected swabs from the throat, vagina, or rectum) are simply obtained and analyzed with new highly accurate nucleic acid (DNA) amplification assays.

Is gonorrhea curable?

Yes.

Is gonorrhea treatable?

Yes, 100 percent cure rate* with a single dose of two medications:

Ceftriaxone 250 intramuscular injection plus azithromycin 1 gram orally one time

Two medications are used simultaneously to lower the possibility of resistant gonorrhea. However, this approach is not fool proof. In just the last several years, resistance to azithromycin has increased from 1 to 4 percent of all gonorrhea strains tested. Three cases of gonorrhea resistant to ceftriaxone have also been documented. If combined resistance became widespread, it would be a world-wide disaster.

A lot of patients ask if they can drink on the antibiotics: No, not if you're going to get so drunk you end up with the same partner. For those antibiotics, alcohol use does not usually make one sick.

*As noted above, the first ever superbug gonorrhea resistant to ceftriaxone and azithromycin was reported in an Englishman who had a sexual encounter in SE Asia in 2018, so the cure rate has to be dropped to 99.99 percent. For the record, he was apparently cured with an expensive intravenous antibiotic.

What are my chances of catching gonorrhea?

Gonorrhea is uber infectious. Yes, you can get it if you have sex in the back seat of a cab. But what I'm really trying to say is that of all the STDs, gonorrhea is the most infectious. Gonorrhea is twice as infectious as syphilis and 750 times more infectious than HIV or HSV!

An infected male will pass on the bacteria about 60 percent of the time per act of vaginal intercourse and 85 percent per act of rectal intercourse. An infected woman will pass gonorrhea to a man 25 percent of the time per act of vaginal intercourse (a man has less exposed mucous membranes). Mouth-to-penis oral sex (60 percent) is far riskier than mouth-to-vagina (2 percent). Mouth to mouth can also occur but the percent risk is not known.

Your chances are contracting gonorrhea are higher in urban regions of lower socio-economic Southeastern states due to higher rates of infection, increased opportunity for sexual contacts, and poor access to timely treatment. New cases per year are 30 times higher in Mississippi than in Maine (246 per 100,000 compared with 8 per 100,000).

Gonorrhea prevention

Awareness is prevention

STD prevention programs have historically emphasized the ABCs of safe sex - with apathetic results.

A. Abstinence. Teens involved in abstinence-only campaigns do not benefit. Decreased vaginal STD rates are more than offset by increased oral and rectal STD rates. (Teens live by the Bill Clinton oral-sex-is-not-sex mantra.) Fully 88 percent of teens who pledged abstinence in middle and high school still engaged in non-vaginal sexual acts — and the contacts tended to be riskier in part due to insufficient education.

**Wake up Utah! Let me repeat.
Abstinence education is part
of the STD problem, not the solution.**

B. Be Faithful. Hard to find fault here, but realistically, not a mainstream trait in any known part of the world. Also, there is no evidence that on a public policy level, campaigns of this sort work.

C. Condoms. Especially helpful for gonorrhea. But while teens use condoms only 50 - 60 percent of the time, as adolescents age, condom use drops even more. Additionally, condoms can break, be misused, or fall off up to 20 percent of the time.

Risk factors: residence in Southeast states, late summer, early age of onset sexual activity, unmarried, past history of gonorrhea, illicit drug use, sex worker, and MSM.

Low grade, nonspecific feelings—don't ignore. Perhaps as many as 40 percent of those with silent gonorrhea really have subtle clinical findings. Education is key. Clues of atypical gonorrhea take many forms: Discharge, urinary discomfort, between cycle bleeding, heavy periods or pain with intercourse. Also, be aware STDs often travel in pairs! If you have a new case of chlamydia, Trich or HSV, don't forget to test for gonorrhea too.

Obviously, women more than men have symptom-free infections and are at risk for more long-term complication from slowly festering infections. If you have funky symptoms, don't live in denial! One study of folks presenting to an STD clinic noted that 40 percent of men and 50 percent of woman continued to have sexual activity despite suspicious urinary and vaginal complaints.

Treatment is prevention

1. Persons with symptoms often continue sex if not told of STD exposure, so tell all partners from the past 60 days to get treated.

2. Expedited partner treatment — getting extra medicine (or prescriptions) from the doctor to give to recent partners. CDC recommends partner treatment and it's now legal in all states!

Prophylaxis is prevention

1. Avoid sex for seven days after treatment.

2. Avoid sex with partner until seven days after he or she completes treatment.

3. Meningococcal B vaccination. Three studies show 30 percent protective effect against gonorrhea.

4. Urinating after sex in one military study was about 30 to 50 percent effective at reducing STD risk.

Protection is prevention

1. Condoms. both male and female.

2. Douching after sex associated with bad outcomes — not a good idea.

CHAPTER 15
Chlamydia — Gonorrhea Lite

Chlamydia is the planet's most common bacterial STD. It's also the most frequently mispronounced (cla-mid-ee-a) and misspelled. If you are sexually active, have multiple partners and use condoms lackadaisically, the odds are high you will get chlamydia once — or multiple times — and quickly learn the correct chlamydia pronunciation and spelling.

Chlamydia has been around forever, but in the old days, all penile drips were diagnosed as gonorrhea. When gonorrhea could finally be isolated and fully treated in the 1940s, doctors were surprised to see cases of persistent urethral discharge. Out of gonorrhea's centuries-old shadow emerged gonorrhea negative "non-specific" urethritis — mostly chlamydia.

Today, chlamydia is the bacterial gorilla in the room: four times more common than gonorrhea. Chlamydial infections and complications generally mirror gonorrhea but chlamydia has fewer physical signs and less intense symptoms. Chlamydia is gonorrhea lite.

But don't let chlamydia's "gonorrhea lite" moniker fool you. Chlamydia is responsible for more scarring and long-term complications than the much more aggressive, symptomatic gonorrhea. Why? Chlamydia's infrequent symptoms means many individuals remain unaware – permitting occult infections to smolder undetected and untreated in the reproductive tubes.

How many are infected (chlamydia prevalence)?

In the U.S., 1.8 million persons have Chlamydia. The percentage of women and men infected (3 percent) is slightly lower than worldwide averages but the rates are quite high in certain populations, i.e., 11 percent in young military men, 15 percent and 20 percent in STD clinic male and female patients, up to 5 percent of pregnant patients and as many as a fourth of some Inuit or native American women.

World-wide, there are 130,000,000 chlamydia carriers. No, that's not a typo, it's really 130 million. More females than males (4.2 percent vs. 2.7 percent) carry this STD because women tend to have less telltale symptoms than men and spontaneous cures take longer.

How many get new infections each year (incidence)?

There were 1.7 million reported (to county health departments) American cases in 2017 – an increase of 5 percent compared with 2016.

Estimates are that 2.9 million Americans get chlamydia each year as many cases go unreported. (They're treated confidentially in a private doctor's office.) Chlamydia is much more common in those less than 25 years old. Some call it an adolescent intern STD! The cervix (opening to the uterus) of teens and young women is not fully matured and probably more susceptible to infection.

Chlamydia: How do you get it?

Chlamydia bacteria readily gains entry through human mucous membranes. It is specially adapted to live in the outermost cells covering moist mucous membranes, which are rich in essential vitamins and amino acids that chlamydia cannot synthesize but desperately craves.

So, no surprise, chlamydia is very infectious via vaginal, oral, and rectal intercourse. Chlamydia can also be passed during childbirth. It can't live outside the human body for long and is not transmitted via toilet seats or dirty towels.

Chlamydia: First warning signs

After a one to three-week incubation, 30 percent of infected women notice new vaginal discharge, urinary discomfort, or abnormal vaginal bleeding. Half of infected men recognize scant, thin, penile discharge or burning with urination. Given the paucity of symptoms, the first warning sign may be a text, usually from the male partner because men, much more likely than woman, recognize early urinary symptoms.

"How r u feeling"? Your recent partner asks.

"When i p something doesn't feel right" with a sad-eyed emoji or *"Urine test off - something called cla mid ee a,"* followed by a repeating row of tearful and sick-faced emojis.

Women: Please don't get mad when a partner contacts you with the "just got diagnosed with chlamydia" news. Yes, it's possible he may have gone outside your relationship without your express written consent, but at least he had the balls to notify you. Many men don't — and that would put you at considerable risk of a damaging occult infection. Also, always keep an open mind. This chlamydia infection may have originated with you! You might have contacted chlamydia years ago and the infection persisted inside you with no symptoms.

Chlamydia: Natural history if you don't treat

Next time you boast "I've never had an STD", remember this bug has zero recognizable pelvic symptoms in 70 percent of infected women and 50 percent of infected men. About 130 million people worldwide wouldn't be walking around with this infection if it were easy to self-diagnose!

Lack of symptoms is a curse; indolent chlamydial infections still can inflame and scar delicate reproductive organs, sometimes to the point of endangering the safe passage of a fertilized egg from ovary to uterus implantation. Furthermore, by disrupting the mucous membrane integrity, untreated chlamydia can increase the chance of getting (or giving) HIV by up to five-fold. Thankfully, chlamydia in most cases is a self-limiting disease: The vast majority of undetected cases spontaneously burn out and resolve after a year.

However, about 10 to 20 percent of the time, chlamydia causes permanent damage by inflaming and scarring uterine, tubal, and intra-abdominal surfaces. This may or may not elicit pelvic pain. Infertility from gummed-up tubes or potentially life-threatening ectopic (tubal) pregnancies may present later when the chlamydia has long departed. Also, it appears chlamydia infections and inflammation of the fallopian tubes increases ovarian cancer risk two-fold. This alone could translate to 2,000 additional deadly ovarian cancers every year.

Guys can get a chlamydia wakeup call when a testicle abruptly starts throbbing for no apparent reason. Male-based infertility–scarred epididymal tubes that carry the sperm out the testicles is less common than the female counterpart. Both sexes can get symptomatic-throat (mild ache) and rectal (urge to defecate with only mucous or bloody discharge) infections but typically chlamydia in these locations remains silent. Rarely, chlamydia makes the immune system go awry, resulting in painful arthritis, pain on urination and pink eye.

Like gonorrhea, chlamydia is a huge concern at childbirth. As many as 5 percent of expecting moms are infected, heightening the risk of a preterm birth and/or low birth weight infant. Without routine prenatal screening of pregnant moms, about 60 to 70 percent of exposed newborns (as many as one in 25 babies) silently acquire chlamydia at birth, placing them at risk for blindness or pneumonia.

Chlamydia: How to diagnose:

Thank God for the new DNA tests for chlamydia! It's a world simpler and far more accurate than what I used to do just several years ago — namely torturing patients by twisting a cotton Q Tip up the urethra. Now the patient just leaves a urine specimen – or if exposure dictates, a self-collected vaginal, throat or rectal swab.

Easy Peesy!

Some doctors continue to advise first morning urines as the best specimens for chlamydia detection, but with these amazing DNA tests, the timing of specimen collection no longer really matters. If chlamydia is present, the test will find it. Immediately request a chlamydia test if you have:

1. plans to get pregnant.
2. pregnancy complications.
3. discomfort (e.g., burning or tingling) on urination.
4. penile or vaginal discharge.
5. nagging pelvic pain.
6. abnormal vaginal bleeding.
7. rectal pain, discharge, or blood.

Yearly tests for:

1. sexually active individuals with new or multiple partners.
2. use social media to arrange casual sexual encounters.
3. infrequent or inconsistent condom use.
4. have sex under the influence of drugs or alcohol.
5. past chlamydia positive (reinfection in first year as high as 30 percent).
6. sexually active non-monogamous MSM (quarterly).
7. all sexually active persons under age 25 years.

Is chlamydia curable?

Yes, 100 percent.

Is chlamydia treatable?

Yes.

Azithromycin 1 gram, one oral dose
or
Doxycycline 100 mg, twice a day x 7 day

Azithromycin is the super convenient first choice. Doxycycline is cheaper than azithromycin and is superior for anal chlamydial infection but it's contraindicated in pregnancy (discolors the baby's teeth) and has more possible side effects (nausea, sun sensitivity).

With either choice, don't have sex for seven days after the first dose. Also make sure recent partners have been treated. Your partners may choose treatment by their own trusted physician, however, "expedited treatment" — giving partners appropriate antibiotics without a face-to-face visit — is now recognized as ethically sound and more medically effective. It's also now legal in all states.

A moderate amount of alcohol with the antibiotics is OK. Just please don't get so inebriated you end up having sex before the seven-day "hold" is up. Pharmacists tell everyone these antibiotics may render birth control pills subtly less effective but that's baloney. There is no evidence this is true (except for anti-tuberculosis drugs like rifampin).

Once treated, it is important to get tested again in 3 months. Not because the medication did not work but because the most consistent predictor of a chlamydial infection is a past chlamydial infection. About 20 percent of men and women who had chlamydia will get it again within the next 3 months.

What Are My Chances of Catching Chlamydia?

Chlamydia is extremely communicable — at or just below the level of gonorrhea. It's six hundred and twenty-five-fold more transmittable than HIV. One episode of vaginal sex with a chlamydia-infected male partner equals a one-in-two chance of the female getting infected. Like gonorrhea, almost twice as many women as men have chlamydia, but men are twice as infectious.

Surprisingly, if you catch chlamydia, like most bacterial STDs, you get little if any immunity. These bacteria are able to change their outer walls over time enabling the bacteria to constantly look different, thereby avoiding the body's usually highly efficient memory immune cells, which search and destroy bacteria and viruses they've seen before. Partly due to this lack of immunity and partly due to repeat contact with former partners or similar partners in your sexual network, there's a crazy high 20 percent chance of getting a repeat infection within 3 months. Beware!

Chlamydia prevention

Awareness is prevention

Learn how to pronounce (cla-mid-ee-a) and spell chlamydia. Recognize its suspicious symptoms too. Understand chlamydia frequently lacks symptoms – get regular testing if you have "high-risk" behavior.

Treatment is prevention

Test and treat early. Stop sexual activity if suspicious symptoms exist to minimize transmission (currently, many don't) and expedite the notification and treatment of partner(s) within the last 60 days.

Let's be honest. There was a record 2.3 million reported cases in the U.S. last year of gonorrhea, syphilis and chlamydia - and probably several million more unreported cases! Why are we doing such an abysmal job of controlling these simply-treated bacterial diseases? Answer — Lack of education/awareness together with a disjointed health system and doctors insisting on covering their collective asses — (and not reporting infections to County health departments) even when the end result is more disease.

STD patients aren't thrilled (understandably) about naming recent partners to the public health department, allowing county employees to contact recent partners making sure everyone exposed gets the proper antibiotics. But now, billions of online matches with estimates of anonymous first-date sex approaching 50 percent has rendered this old school STD control strategy nearly impossible.

Doctors aren't thrilled to hand their chlamydia patient extra scripts (or better extra packets of antibiotic pills) to treat unseen partners. Doctors have been brainwashed since medical school. They believe for ethical, quality of care, and legal reasons, they must see every patient face-to-face. This has advantages, but demanding exposed partners make doctor visits is too expensive, too embarrassing, and frankly ineffective! Americans with chlamydia have voted with their feet. They far prefer to deliver appropriate antibiotics to their partners themselves, although contacting ex's can be a struggle when phone numbers go "cold." Interestingly, for years gynecologists have "blindly" treated partners of woman with trichomonas, but that's a low-level, unemotional, easily treated disease.

In 2001, as a direct result of Dr. K's undeniable persistence, the California Department of Health Services took a big step to help doctors too fearful of legal liability to do the right thing (i.e. pass out packets of antibiotics blindly for all partners of the original case). They supported a change in the state law. The law now permits doctors to give patients treatment for their partners for chlamydial and/or gonococcal infection. If your doctor is not offering that, it may be time to educate him or her!

Prophylaxis is prevention

The ABCs:

Abstention: This option is best on paper only. Promoting abstinence is fantasy. Several research studies have concluded its outright harmful. High school students taught abstinence actually have higher STD and unwanted pregnancy rates!

Imagine teaching a kid to ride a bike and telling him the best way to be safe riding a bike is *not to ride one!* C'mon dad, get real!

Be faithful: In a mutually monogamous relationship with a tested partner. Hard to find too much fault here, but it takes a while for many of us to find that perfect steady partner.

Condoms: When used correctly, (i.e. no breakage, no slipping off at the conclusion of intercourse, no non-penetrative foreplay where secretions spread with fingers) are extremely effective.

CHAPTER 16
Mycoplasma: STD Rookie of the Year

Breaking news: *Mycoplasma genitalium* has just been named STD rookie of the year. Microbiologists only confirmed its status as an actual STD several years ago, and already it's entered the top venereal disease list at No. 4, just behind chlamydia!

Mycoplasma was identified in human genital secretions back in the 1980s, but because cultures were unreliable (and took up to six months to grow), it was nearly impossible to track these tiny intracellular bacteria and see if they were disease causing. With the recent advent of DNA testing, researchers instantly discovered that all along, mycoplasma was up to no good! Literally under our noses, it was causing millions of chlamydia-like urethral, cervical, and fallopian tube infections. To complicate matters, mycoplasma is often resistant to the antibiotics used for chlamydia, gonorrhea, or trichomonas. So symptomatic or not, in many instances mycoplasma festers in the genital tract undiagnosed and untreated, poised to inflame the urethra, cervix, or fallopian tubes, contributing to America's rampant infertility problem.

In America today, one in nine young couples are infertile! Spoiler alert: a real-life *Handmaid's Tale*?

How many are infected (prevalence) and how many get new infections each year (incidence)?

There are no good studies yet, but it appears to be as common as chlamydia, so our best estimates are about 2.8 million new cases of mycoplasma in the U.S. each year.

Mycoplasma: How do you get it?

You get mycoplasma by exposure during condom-less sex to infected penile, vaginal, or rectal secretions.

Mycoplasma: First warning signs

Most persons recently infected with mycoplasma have no suspicious symptoms whatsoever. Typically, 7 to 10 days after infection, 30 percent of people have symptoms: Males can complain of burning with urination or a thin, slightly milky penile (or rectal) discharge; females can notice unusual vaginal discharge, pain with intercourse, or intercourse-related vaginal bleeding.

Mycoplasma's natural history if you don't treat

Best case, untreated mycoplasma remains silent and after an uneventful year the infection burns out without a trace. On the other hand, mycoplasma can start out low key with trivial or no signs, then form abscesses causing painful inflammation and permanent scarring inside genital structures. Occasional complications in males include: testicular pain and swelling, urethral strictures and chronic discomfort with urination or ejaculation, and even infertility. In females, complications include pelvic inflammatory disease, unexplained chronic pelvic pain, infertility, and/or pregnancy difficulties like miscarriage or preterm birth. Mycoplasma also scars the fallopian tubes and may cause tubal pregnancy when the fertilized egg cannot make it through the blocked passageway from the ovaries into the uterus. About 2 percent of all pregnancies (80,000 per year) occur in the tubes. Tubal pregnancies can be life threatening. There are about 1,000 maternal deaths yearly in the U.S. About 15 percent (150 deaths) are due to tubal pregnancies. On this basis, every year mycoplasma, chlamydia, and gonorrhea are each responsible for up to 50 deaths.

Mycoplasma diagnosis:

Just several years ago, mycoplasma genital infections were impossible to prove. There was no reliable test.

Diagnosis based on symptoms? Most mycoplasma infections cause no symptoms.

Diagnosis based on urinary and vaginal symptoms? Doctors will first blame gonorrhea, chlamydia, Trichomonas, yeast or bacterial vaginosis (BV).

Diagnose it for persistent urinary or vaginal symptoms resistant to "usual" STD antibiotics? Doctors should have, but often didn't.

Then in 2016 — drum roll please — the DNA mycoplasma test arrived. This test is now available in all commercial laboratories as a stand-alone urine test or alternatively a swab from urethral, rectal or vaginal secretions.

The underfunded CDC is struggling to meet the daunting challenges of resurgent chlamydia, gonorrhea, and syphilis. It can barely summon the resources to educate doctors, much less the general public, about the new bad boy on the street, mycoplasma. As a result, major doctor associations like the American College of Gynecologists still instruct their members not to test or treat for mycoplasma. They are out of date. Same goes for the majority of doctors unaware of the studies proving the existence of this potentially troublesome disease and unaware of the new accurate DNA test.

Doctors H and K Recommend:
If you want a *complete* STD check,
for now, it's up to you. Request a
mycoplasma DNA test be included.

If you have a mycoplasma infection diagnosed, all past partners over the last two months should be offered treatment. If residual symptoms remain, retest for mycoplasma and other potential co-infecting STDs.

Is mycoplasma curable?

Yes, absolutely. However, like gonorrhea, mycoplasma bacteria are adept at figuring out how to resist certain antibiotics, so treatment must be carefully selected. For example, antibiotics used to treat chlamydia and gonorrhea often are ineffective against mycoplasma. There should be new technology available soon to tell doctors what the best antibiotic is to treat mycoplasma infection.

Mycoplasma treatment:

Moxifloxacin 400 mg by mouth for 10 days (success rates vary from 70% - 100%)

or

Azithromycin 1.5-2.5 gram by mouth one time (a wide range of success, from 40 - 85%)

or

Doxycycline 100 mg twice daily for 7 days followed by Azithromycin 1.5 gram over 2 days (>90% effective)

Moxifloxacin and doxycycline are not recommended to be used during pregnancy. Moxifloxacin can infrequently cause tendon problems in runners.

Infectivity: What are my chances of catching mycoplasma?

Mycoplasma is very infectious. It's 560-times more contagious than HIV, on par with both gonorrhea and chlamydia. If you have sex with someone with mycoplasma, after one condom-less sexual contact, you have just under a 50 percent chance of getting infected.

If you have multiple partners, and use condoms lackadaisically, it's not "if" but "when" you will get a dose of mycoplasma.

Mycoplasma prevention

Awareness is prevention

Know the facts. Mycoplasma is infectious. Mycoplasma is common. Most doctors do not test for it in their "thorough" STD checks. Mycoplasma can cause substantial genital organ damage leading to infertility or rarely even death.

Mycoplasma is curable — with the right antibiotics — but first, you have to be pro-active and ask about mycoplasma and the correct diagnostic test. For example, Dr. H, will my urine test include the test for mycoplasma? Or, Dr. H. will my vaginal swab test also test for mycoplasma? I heard it is as common as chlamydia and want to be tested.

PS, blame me if the doctor gives you attitude!

Treatment is prevention

Treatment reduces the duration of infection. Therefore, treatment results in fewer people carrying mycoplasma at any given time. Effective and timely treatment is important both for your overall health, to prevent long-term mycoplasma complications like infertility, and for the public health, since fewer people will be infected.

Protection is prevention

Latex (or polyurethane) male or female condoms work. Condoms serve as barriers to the spread of mycoplasma infection. Remember, condoms can hold water or even air (they make great balloons), so they can easily hold or block germs like mycoplasma. However, for condoms to work, they must be used correctly.

CHAPTER 17
Trichomoniasis: The Rodney Dangerfield of STDs

Trichomoniasis — better known simply as "Trich" — is the Rodney Dangerfield of STDs. It's the No. 5 most common STD but it gets no respect.

Caused by the parasite *Trichomonas vaginalis*, it can result in discharge. It can occasionally cause vaginal malodor. It can increase baby mortality. It triples the risk of acquiring HIV. But most people have never heard of this resilient five-tailed parasite. The press is generally uninterested, even given the fact Trich infects over 140 million persons a year worldwide!

Trich flies under the radar because its symptoms are subtle. In fact, 85 percent of infections cause no symptoms at all. And, until very recently, Trich was quite difficult to diagnose.

I certainly will always give Trichomonas vaginalis the respect it deserves. In college, I'll never forget my very first girlfriend sitting me down in her dorm room and informing me her gynecologist had just diagnosed trichomoniasis on a routine GYN exam. She had no symptoms. I had no symptoms. She told me it usually wasn't an STD ("nuns can get it") but that her doctor recommended "just in case," we both take a course of an antibiotic called Flagyl, which could not be taken with any alcohol. I remember initially having doubts, but I really liked this woman, and I just took the medication.

How many people get new Trich infections each year?

1.1 million (U.S.), 140 million (worldwide).

How prevalent is Trich?

In the U.S., 3.1 percent women (2.3 million), (3.2 percent pregnant woman), 1.9 percent men (1.4 million); worldwide: 5.0 percent of women. The prevalence rises with age, number of sex partners, and is more common among African-Americans.

How is Trich contracted?

We now know that essentially all Trich (99 percent) is contracted through vaginal or anal sex.

Up to 1 percent of women with no history of sexual intercourse contract Trich. Yes, nuns can get it. (Whew, she was telling me the truth!) Cases have been documented from sharing contaminated douche nozzles, moist wash-clothes, soiled towels, or possibly Jacuzzis (Dr. K is very skeptical of this), but never from kissing or sharing utensils. It can also be passed from a mother to her baby at birth or even from cryo-bank semen.

What are the first warning signs of Trich?

The first warning sign is zilch: 85 percent of cases have no complaints at all.

Symptomatic men report minor irritation after urination or ejaculation or occasionally a wispy penile discharge leaving a yellow crust (see the White Underwear Test). Symptomatic women report minor burning, discomfort with urination, or a thin yellow to greenish discharge or rarely pelvic pain. Occasionally, Trich can be associated with vaginal malodor.

What is the Trich worst-case scenario if not treated?

Trich can silently loiter inside the reproductive tracts for months or years, especially in women. Best-case scenario: You peacefully co-exist with this wily parasite and after a few months the infection spontaneously resolves. It's unknown what is different in the minority who report symptoms usually one to four weeks after exposure.

However, Trich can cause a chronic discharge. Infection in males can trigger a scant thin discharge, burning, and frequent urination along with perineal (between the scrotum and rectum) pain.

Worse case, inflamed genital tissue associated even with symptom free Trich increases susceptibility to all other STDs. Specifically, it trebles the risk of acquiring HIV. In parts of Africa where the risk of getting HIV is already sky high, by increasing the likelihood of getting HIV, Trich can be lethal!

Trich infestation during pregnancy is a bad actor too. Its credits include preterm delivery, low birth weight, and increased baby mortality. Transmission of trichomoniasis from an infected mother to baby during delivery is rare, but respiratory or genital infection of the newborn is possible.

How is Trich diagnosed?

Back in the day, Trich was a bear to diagnose. The microscope slide test was the best we had! I would stand in the lab as a bewildered resident, stirred vaginal secretions scraped from a speculum into a test tube and then placed a precious drop onto a microscope slide. Then I had to stare for what seemed like hours deep into the microscope searching for a five-tailed Trich to wiggle across the screen.

Doctors now have it easy. They don't have to get anywhere near a microscope! They merely order the Trich DNA test done on a urine (or alternatively on a vaginal swab) which is run in an outside lab. It can accurately diagnose trichomoniasis in over 95 percent of cases.

DOCTORS H AND K SUGGEST:

The White Underwear Test (for men): If in doubt about the presence of discharge - wear a snug pair of white underwear ("tighty whities") to bed.

In the morning, you have your answer.
Crusty off white/yellow/green stains confirm an abnormal discharge.
No frontal stains: You have no discharge.
Thin, water-based "clear" stains are equivocal. Males can have several drops of urine normally escape after urination.

Rarely, black powder (pubic lice droppings) and miniscule white dots (pubic lice eggs) can be seen in your underwear.

Is Trich curable?

Yes, 100 percent.

Is Trich treatable?

Yes, 100 percent.

Metronidazole, 500 mg twice daily for 7 days

But duh! Trich will surface again with repeat exposure to an infected person. Consequently, about 20 percent of folks who have taken a curative antibiotic for trichomoniasis get reinfected within three months. Like with every other STD, you've gotta notify all recent contacts to get them treated.

Metronidazole is okay for pregnant but not breastfeeding women. It's the one drug that when you are on it, you should truly avoid alcohol or risk nausea and stomach upset.

What are my chances of catching Trich?

Pretty high. Your chance of getting it appears to be about 40 percent with a single episode of condom-less sex with an infected partner, but convincing data is lacking.

Now the bookend Trich story. An early scare in Dr. K's life was waking up next to a girl he met during Mardi Gras and upon learning he was a hot shot med student, she asked him to help her interpret a letter she'd just received from the Louisiana Department of Public Health. The letter stated she'd been diagnosed with Trich, needed treatment, and must notify her recent partners. (There was apparently no mention that Louisiana nuns get it!) He wonders to this day if that was her not-so-subtle way of notifying him. He told her how to get treated and that, fortunately at least for him, was the story's end. Since he had used a condom properly he was not exposed and would not get infected. Saved by latex.

But I believe that woman did society a great service. She may have subconsciously influenced his career choice, and we all benefit from his efforts to destigmatize STDs while prioritizing efforts to eradicate them.

Can Trich be prevented?

Condoms effectively reduce Trich transmission, but they are not a total panacea because in the U.S., the failure rate of condoms is estimated to be between 10 and 30 percent — disappointingly high.

Vaginal Irritation, Itching and Discharge			
	Bacterial Vaginosis	**Yeast**	**Trich**
Discharge	thin whitish clings to walls*	thick cottage cheese clings to walls	thick yellow-green frothy
Malodor	fish odor	none	occasional
Itching	unlikely	likely	likely
Urinary pain	unlikely	sometimes	less likely
Testing:			
pH	high	normal	high-normal
microscopic	cells coated with bacteria	budding yeast	mobile Trich increased WBCs
DNA tests	available	none	available
* Vaginal walls			

Table 9

CHAPTER 18
Crabs (Public Lice) — The Dinosaur of STDs

Crabs (pubic lice), tiny six-legged creatures roughly 1/16-inch long with strong crab-like pincers specifically designed to attach to coarse pubic hair (Figure 30), have been crawling around human loins since the beginning of mankind. Pubic lice remnants have been discovered in hair of archeological remains from 18 centuries ago. DNA analysis suggests crabs — and cavemen with scratchy crotches — coexisted 5.6 million years ago.

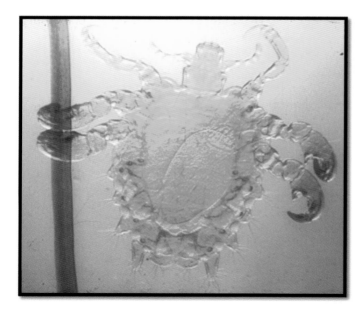

Figure 30 - Pubic Louse. Magnified crab with two pinchers firmly attached to pubic hair

Amazingly, after prospering on the earth for over 5 million years, in a few short decades, crab infestations have dramatically decreased. Back in the day, crabs were far and away the No. 1 STD I treated. I'd see at least one a day in the early '90s. Today, I cannot remember one case I've seen in the last year or two! What happened? With the explosion of online dating matches, sex is certainly not decreasing. In fact, other STDs (chlamydia, gonorrhea, and syphilis) are markedly increasing year after year. Long story short: We're not the same hairy mammal we once were. The unprecedented 96 percent drop in crabs seen in some studies, parallels the near global adaptation of extreme hair removal techniques, especially the "Brazilian."

Are crabs on the verge of extinction? Are pubic lice the dinosaur of STDs? How many are newly infected (incidence)?

Use of anti-crab medication in the 1990s suggested as many as 3 million pubic lice infestations in the U.S. per year. The current incidence is less than 120,000.

Crabs: How do you get it?

Crabs are spread via sexual contact. In rare instances, the infestation begins after contact with toilet seats, clothing, bed sheets, and dirty towels used by an infected person. Pets fortunately do not get pubic lice. They play no role in transmission.

First warning signs of crabs:

The first symptom is pubic itchiness approximately five to seven days after the initial exposure. Sometimes, the crab bites do not elicit an allergic response and itching never occurs. Rarely, individuals first see black residue (lice droppings) and miniscule white eggs in their underwear.

Natural history of crabs if you don't treat:

Once adult crabs are transferred via sexual contact, they instantly go to work procreating! The females lay four eggs per day over their entire one-month life. (Pubic lice die in a day if isolated from the human body). The pubic lice eggs hatch in about 5 to 10 days, in part based on the body's heat. The baby crabs require frequent blood meals as they mature in a little over a week into mature egg laying adults. To feed, the crabs stab through the skin, pump saliva filled with an anti-clotting chemical into the skin puncture sites to ensure a good drop of blood can exit, and lastly suction the blood into its digestive tract, engorging the body.

Crabs do not transmit disease. They do elicit a skin allergic reaction in the human host resulting in incessant itching. When skin is scratched hard enough, especially with long fingernails, bacterial boils or localized skin infection can result.

Diagnosis of crabs:

The diagnosis is made by the visual identification of pubic lice and/or their eggs (nits).

An examiner can see pubic lice (usually moving) and their eggs with the naked eye — at least up until the age of 45 when reading glasses are necessary — but some doctors use a magnifying glass for difficult cases. Self-diagnosing pubic lice can be more difficult; You are an extra two feet away and it's difficult to identify lice or their eggs if you haven't ever seen them before.

Are crabs curable?

Yes.

Treatment of crabs:

1% permethrin cream rinse. Apply once to affected regions, rinse off after 10 minutes, take soap and water shower, and towel dry.
or
pyrethins with piperonyl butoxide. Apply once to affected regions, rinse off after 10 minutes, take soap and water shower, and towel dry.

These products are all off patent and can be purchased generic now, so they are much less expensive than before. Twice as much is not twice as effective so use exactly according to package instructions. Both these medication options are OK in pregnant and lactating women.

Both treatments are now available over-the-counter. My all-time favorite brand name drug is the pubic lice drug *BARC: crab spelled backward!* Who could ever forget a name like that?

Crabs rarely present on eyebrow, eyelash, beard, mustache, chest or armpit hair. Never use these products for eyelash infestations. Occasionally some strains are resistant to these medications; your doctor will discuss the safest second-line treatments.

Following treatment, most nits (crab eggs) will still be attached to hair shafts. Nits may be removed with fingernails or by a fine-toothed comb. We suggest you consider removing all pubic hair by shaving if crabs are documented. Put on fresh underwear and clothing after treatment. To kill any lice or nits that might remain on clothing, towels, or bedding (which could live up to several days), machine wash in hot cycle and machine dry all items used in the two to three days before treatment. Sometimes, you can put all the laundry in the wash in the 10 minutes the medication is soaking in. Items that cannot be laundered can be dry-cleaned or stored in a sealed plastic bag for two weeks. Inform all sex partners from the previous 30 days. Search for live crabs on the tenth day after treatment when remaining eggs would normally hatch. Also screen for other STDs.

DOCTORS H AND K SUGGEST:

If crabs are documented, treat appropriately (above),
then remove all pubic hair (by shaving) to eliminate
the chance of residual crab eggs. Remember, hold off on sex
with unknown partner for 48 hours after shaving.

Itching can persist long after all pubic lice and eggs are killed. Skin allergic reactions can take a week or more to cool off. Scratch marks characteristically itch during the healing phase and some patients freak out just at the thought of lice (parasitophobia).

Yes, to reiterate, it's definitely possible to itch for psychological reasons. I saw a whole floor of nurses (who together had bathed an uncooperative homeless person) start madly itching after learning the man had both crabs and scabies.

Infectivity - What are my chances of catching crabs?

Experience throughout human history suggests pubic lice are extremely infectious, but no exact scientific data exists. Pubic lice are programmed to attach to coarse pubic hair, but they can crawl (slowly, perhaps no more than four inches per day) and will occasionally travel to chest or armpits regions. When pubic hair is removed, infectivity drops dramatically. Beard, eyelash, and eyebrow hair may become infected from oral sex but these hair types are not the pubic louse's natural habitat.

Prevention of crabs:

Illuminate your pubic hair. Crabs hate bright light and will frantically try to get away! OK, this weird science fact is not exactly practical!

Better yet, if you've been infected, consider complete pubic hair removal — and hold off on sex for at least two days after hair removal.

CHAPTER 19

Bacterial Vaginosis: Pubic Nuisance

If you have unusual vaginal discharge, malodor, or just vague vaginal discontent, bacterial vaginosis (BV) is the most likely suspect.

Lactobacillus bacteria are the predominant inhabitant of the normal vaginal microbial ecosystem, pumping out lactic acid and hydrogen peroxide, which keeps the vaginal surfaces acidic at pH < 4.5, thereby keeping other microbes in check. Normal "physiologic" vaginal discharge consists of scant estrogen-dependent cervical secretions plus sloughed vaginal cells and normal bacteria.

But this environment is easily disrupted. Intercourse with multiple partners, obesity, smoking, and vaginal douching can cause a microorganism overgrowth condition. Healthy vaginal lactobacillus is replaced by finicky bacteria with weird names, like Gardnerella, Prevotella, Atobium and Mobiluncus. Not only do these bothersome microbes secrete enzymes creating excess mucous, they also fashion funky smells by releasing eerily named volatile gases (e.g. putrescine, cadaverine, trimethylamine) as byproducts of their unique metabolism.

Half the time, BV shows up as a slightly fish-smelling milky thin white vaginal discharge. The other half of the time, there are either no symptoms or symptoms so mild that the woman has finally "given up" and accepted them as "normal."

BV is a sex-related disease:
1. It can crop up after a new male partner.
2. It can crop up after a new female partner.
3. Condoms seem to lower BV risk.
4. The disease hallmark is finding overgrowth of Gardnerella or other unusual bacteria in the face of diminished levels of vaginal lactobacillus.
5. Metronidazole pills or clindamycin vaginal cream make it go away.
6. Non-sexually active women are rarely affected.

BV is not a classic sexually transmitted disease (STD):

1. Though the exposed male partner can carry one or more of the atypical BV-associated bacteria, males get no symptoms and no disease.
2. Furthermore, treating the male partner doesn't affect the women's chance of BV cure – or future recurrence.

Prevalence:

Surprising numbers of sexually active woman have BV — up to 30 percent — half with and half without obvious symptoms.

Unfortunately, some practitioners shoulder-shrug when women voice subtle discharge and odor complaints. These docs believe BV symptoms are trivial and diagnosis and treatment are questionable. This pervasive misconception results in delayed and often inadequate treatment.

Diagnosis:

1) BV discharge: homogeneous, milky thin discharge that smoothly coats vaginal walls.
2) A fishy odor, especially when a potassium hydroxide solution is mixed with vaginal discharge, i.e. the infamous whiff test.
3) Vaginal discharge has a pH greater than 4.5 (vaginal pH is normally acidic with a pH less than 4.5).
4) Greater than 20 percent of cells in vaginal discharge on microscopic examination are clue cells. (This is over-the-head technical but for the docs and microbiologists out there, clue cells are vaginal epithelial cells studded with adherent coccobacilli bacteria.)
5) Gardnerella DNA test: helpful if Gardnerella detected but since many cases of BV do not have Gardnerella overgrowth a negative or normal test is not that helpful.

According to researchers, you have BV if three of the first four items above are present (the Amstel criteria) but in the real-world, docs begin treatment if:

1. You have a milky thin discharge with or without malodor.
2. Your urine DNA tests for GC, chlamydia, mycoplasma and Trich tests are negative.
3. You have no yeast overgrowth. (Yeast discharge is usually a thicker "cottage cheese" consistency, but it can sometime be thin, making visual differentiation from BV impossible.)
4. BV DNA test is positive (a new test, recently available at commercial laboratories)

Complications of untreated BV:

Women with BV are more likely to get STDs, especially HIV, gonorrhea chlamydia and herpes. They also are more likely to get pelvic inflammatory disease or complications after terminations or gynecological surgery.

Pregnant women: Be on the lookout for subtle BV signs! Women with a prior preterm birth are at high risk for repeat preterm delivery, late miscarriage, and adverse outcomes in the neonate but benefit from BV treatment if testing is positive. Either oral metronidazole or intravaginal clindamycin are safe for baby and comforting for mother.

One word of caution: It's tricky discerning normal/physiologic vaginal discharge (which increases in pregnancy) and vaginal yeast overgrowth (also common place during pregnancy) from BV discharge. Currently the detection and treatment of asymptomatic BV in pregnancy is controversial. One study showed more harm than good, another showed decreased risk of premature labor, so the obstetricians I know treat all pregnancy-related BV.

Treatment:

Metronidazole 500 mg orally twice a day for 7 days
or
Clindamycin cream 2%, one full applicator (5 g) intravaginally at bedtime for 7 days
and
Stop tobacco. There is a two-to-three-fold increased chance of BV in cigarette smokers.

Alcohol and metronidazole don't mix, so avoid booze while on this antibiotic and for three days thereafter or risk igniting chemo-level nausea and vomiting. This drug is notable for killing the overgrowing bad bacteria but not affecting the essential good lactobacillus strains.

Clindamycin cream is oil-based and can compromise the integrity of latex condoms and diaphragms. Use a different form of contraception during and five days after use.

Probiotic preparations or intravaginal non-medical lactobacillus (or yogurt) have not worked and are not recommended. Triple sulfa intravaginal creams are not effective treatment for BV.

Sex partners need not be notified or treated. Follow-up visits are unnecessary if symptoms resolve. Unfortunately, recurrent BV is common, so other empiric approaches — like switching to NuvaRing for birth control or monthly metronidazole plus, an anti-yeast treatment — are occasionally needed.

.

CHAPTER 20
Urinary Tract Infections (UTIs): Adolescent Initiation

A first urinary tract infection (UTI) can be outright scary.

Often a few days after sex, perplexing symptoms come out of nowhere: a pepper spray urination sting, an out of body urgency to pee, an urge to go seemingly every five minutes and sometimes bloody or weirdly malodorous urine.

First timers freak out, logically fearing they have contracted a raging STD. UTIs are the most common bacterial infection in the U.S. so this story is repeated over and over.

How many women of child bearing age will get a UTI?

By age 24, a third of all American women will have had at least one bout of these attention-grabbing symptoms — urinary pain, frequency, urgency, sometimes plus blood in the urine, and increased night urination — all resolved by a few days of antibiotics. Half of all American women will have a UTI at some point in their lives. Unfortunately, once you join this club, you are prone to get repeated UTIs.

UTIs are sex-related diseases:

1. Intercourse tends to "massage" vaginal bacteria up the urethra into the typically sterile bladder — and urine is a pretty good culture medium for many bacteria, especially in pregnancy.
2. UTIs tend to appear two days after intercourse, about the time it takes for rapidly dividing bacteria to gain a foothold into the wall of the bladder.
3. UTIs are especially common with new or infrequent sex partners. In fact, UTI's are so common two days after weddings that there's a name for it: *Honeymoon Cystitis*.

4. As many as 50 percent of women with discomfort on urination after "good sex" actually have local trauma, not a UTI as the cause of their complaints.

5. Females get thirty-fold more UTIs than men because of anatomical differences: the distance from the tip of the urethra to the bladder is considerably longer in men (inches) compared with women (a fraction of an inch).

UTIs are not sexually transmitted diseases (STDs):

1. Using condoms and spermicides do not lower UTI risk. In fact, they may actually increase the rate due to increased friction.

2. Though the exposed male partner can carry one or more of the bacteria known to cause UTIs, males rarely get UTIs (0.1 percent per year for ages 18-50) and do not seem to be source of UTIs in women.

3. Treatment of male partner doesn't in any way affect the women's chance of UTI cure — or future recurrence.

Risky signs for pre-menopausal woman:

Sexual activity (especially multiple encounters after an abstinence period), obesity, having a mom who gets UTIs, diabetes, use of spermicides, and recent antibiotic use all increase the risk of getting UTIs. Next to sex, obesity is the worst offender; markedly elevated body fat increases UTI risk four-fold.

Complications if no treatment:

Infrequently, UTI ascends up from the bladder via the ureter to cause a kidney infection. This potentially dangerous complication that can lead to life-threatening sepsis is signaled by flank pain between the bottom of the wing bone (scapula) and the waist, fever, and general malaise.

Old wives' tales:

Your mom told you wiping back to front, not voiding after sex, and douching all caused UTIs, but there's no scientific evidence that mom's pearls of wisdom are true.

Diagnosis:

1. Classic discomfort and burning on urination and having to urgently pee very frequently.

2. White blood cells (WBC) seen in the urine via microscopic exam.

3. Positive urine culture, i.e. growth of a significant number of bacteria from the urine. (Urine is supposed to be sterile.)

Treatment:

Amoxicillin 250 mg three times a day for 3 days
or
Bactrim DS one tab twice a day for three days
and
Phenazopyridine Hydrochloride (over the counter urethral numbing agent), one pill twice a day for 2 days; if urinary burning severe.

Cranberry products: lots of conflicting information, most of it negative, on whether they work. Please don't depend on them.

The urine culture returns in 48 - 72 hours. Assuming the correct antibiotic was originally given, no more than the three originally prescribed days of antibiotics is usually required. If the microbe is resistant to the initially prescribed antibiotic (less than 10 percent of the time), the appropriate drug is prescribed.

Treatment for recurrent UTIs:

Push fluids:

This safe, cost effective and common-sense approach to UTI's has just been scientifically shown to work! Women with more than 3 UTIs per year were studied. Those able to consume an extra 1.5 liter per day (2 extra cups of water three times a day) had a 50 percent reduction in the number of urinary infections. Presumably the additional fluid flushes out the urine collecting system, literally diluting or washing away harmful bacteria. Please try to skip bottled water and hydrate with local tap water, saving money and sparing the environment from extra plastic trash! Yes, the Flint Michigan water situation was a shocking breakdown in the oversight of our most precious resource, but rest assured tap water is extensively tested and safe throughout the United States.

Antibiotics:

   a. Low dose continuous antibiotics. (Low-dose trimethoprim/ sulfamethoxazole has been tried for up to five years.)
   b. An antibiotic within two hours of intercourse.
   c. Self-starting a three-day antibiotic course, the minute UTI warning signs crop up. A urine culture is not necessary because after UTI self-diagnosis, there is about a 90 percent concordance between self-diagnosis and urine culture in woman with repeated UTIs.

Each of the above treatment options is quite successful. Unfortunately, when antibiotic prophylaxis is discontinued, women revert to their previous frequency of UTI.

CHAPTER 21
Yeast

Yeast infections, also known as candidiasis, are more than a ho-hum everyday nuisance. Although the number of yeast is not directly related to the extent of symptoms, when yeast overgrows, any of the following at best barely tolerable symptoms can present: itching at outer edge vagina, white "cottage cheese" discharge, outer vaginal discomfort with urination, vaginal soreness, swelling, redness, and pain with intercourse.

Woman typically self-treat with over-the-counter anti-fungal creams available at the corner (or online) pharmacy but self-diagnosis is an iffy proposition: Only half of these women actually have a yeast infection. Purported "yeast symptoms" better resolve in three days or you should get suspicious something else is going on.

As previously mentioned, lactobacillus is the predominant inhabitant of the delicate vaginal microbial ecosystem. Small amounts of yeast are also completely normal. Lactobacillus continuously pumps out lactic acid and hydrogen peroxide, which keeps the vagina acidic thereby inhibiting other bothersome microbes. But this environment is easily disrupted in favor of yeast overgrowth, most notably by antibiotics, immunosuppressive drugs including cortisone, diabetes, pregnancy, and even saliva transferred during oral sex. Antibiotics that kill lactobacillus, specifically penicillin, sulfas, and tetracyclines most potently open up territory for the overgrowth of yeast. As luck would have it, metronidazole, the antibiotic used to resolve BV, does not tend to kill the essential good lactobacillus bacteria.

Many women with uncomplicated yeast infections have no discernable precipitating factors.

The number of women currently affected with yeast?

Over three quarters of American woman have had at least one "candida" vaginal infection. Up to 60 percent of pregnant women in their third trimester have vaginal yeast infections. Up to 50 percent of non-pregnant woman may have vaginal yeast detected, but low quantities of yeast can be normal.

Candidiasis is a sex-related disease:

1. Sex can introduce yeast into the vagina. About 10 to 20 percent of men with no abnormal symptoms have yeast colonized on their penis.
2. Receiving oral sex might lead to yeast infections. Roughly 30 percent of healthy people have yeast in their mouth. The introduction of any foreign substance — including saliva, bacteria, and yeast — may be enough to throw off that balance of good germs in the vagina.
3. Elevated estrogen — occurring naturally in pregnancy and from birth control pills (BCPs) — increase risk.

Candidiasis is only rarely an STD:

1. About 10 percent of male sex partners have balanitis, characterized by red patchy areas (and sometimes sores) on the glans of the penis and under the foreskin in conjunction with itching or irritation. These men benefit from treatment with topical antifungal agents to relieve symptoms.
2. Other than above, no partner treatment recommended.
3. No data exist to support the treatment of sex partners of patients with complicated vaginal candidiasis.
4. Frequent sexual activity and having multiple different partners does not increase the risk for vaginal yeast infections.

Diagnosis:

1) Vaginal discharge: thick (can rarely be thin), white, tenacious, "cottage cheese" consistency.
2) Subjective symptoms: exterior itching, redness.
3) Microscopic exam: budding yeast present in vaginal discharge.
4) Culture: positive for yeast species.
5) Vaginal pH: normal.
6) 'Whiff Test': Potassium hydroxide mixed with vaginal discharge is negative – no malodor.

Complications if untreated:

Rarely, the itching from vulvar-vaginal candidiasis can get out of hand, literally, resulting in vulvar swelling, scratch marks, and actual cuts with scabbing. However, the worse part of a yeast infections is the incorrect self-diagnosis.

This often delays treatment and thereby increases complications of other more troublesome causes of vaginal discharge, including BV, gonorrhea, chlamydia. Mycoplasma, or Trich. Remember: Expect the yeast infection to completely resolve in three days with the proper anti-fungal treatment or get suspicious something else is going on.

Treatment:

Miconazole 4% cream 5 g intravaginally daily for 3 days
or
Miconazole 200 mg vaginal suppository, one suppository for 3 days (90% cure rate)
or
Fluconazole 150 mg orally pill in a single dose
or
Miconazole 200 mg vaginal suppository, one suppository for 7 days for pregnant women
or
Miconazole 200 mg vaginal suppository, one suppository for 14 days if the woman is on immunosuppressant or cortisone therapy, if recurrent yeast (may be an unusual strain) or severe swelling and or sores from scratching.

Miconazole cream is an oil-based product that might weaken latex condoms. Fluconazole is prescription medication (except in Mexico) that is quite effective and convenient. Treatment is for those with symptomatic vaginal yeast overgrowth — not for those with vaginal yeast but no symptoms. Acidophilus treatments do not work.

1. Quickie HIV Overview (Chapter 5)

Just three decades ago, human immunodeficiency virus (HIV) was the worst, most terrifying STD the world had ever known. Now HIV is fully treatable and fully preventable. Under certain circumstances, fully treated HIV positive individuals can even have sex without a condom - and not transmit it! (But condom-less sex means the chance of getting gonorrhea, syphilis, chlamydia and other STDs goes way up through!)

In America, the number of new HIV cases is declining, but 39,000 individuals still catch HIV each year, an estimated 1.1 million currently have this lifelong infection and nearly 7,000 still die each year from complications. One half of HIV-infected Americans are either completely unaware they have HIV, not treated or not appropriately treated - these individuals transmit all the new HIV infections. Worldwide, 37 million people currently live with HIV infection — half women and children — the majority undiagnosed or inadequately treated.

If you have HIV infection, antiretroviral medication can fully suppress it, giving you a normal life span and preventing transmission - even when engaging in condom-less oral, vaginal or anal sex.

If you are HIV-uninfected and are contemplating sex with a "high-risk" individual (MSM (men who have sex with men), IV drug user, sex worker or a heterosexual with high-risk partners), consider taking pre-exposure prophylaxis (PrEP) medication to markedly decrease your risk of contracting HIV (over 99 percent effective). If you experience flu-like symptoms several weeks after a "risky" hook-up — or are just concerned you may be in trouble — get a blood test for HIV. Remember, it takes 1 - 3 months for the test to turn positive so be sure to do a follow-up test 3 months later. Alternatively, there is a more expensive genetic test that turns positive in just 10-14 days (HIV RNA blood test, 99 percent accurate).

Bottom line, HIV is no longer a death sentence, so there's no reason to fear getting tested and treated.

HIV Summary

Incidence (new U.S. cases/year):   39,000

Prevalence (total U.S. cases):   1,100,000

Initial symptoms: Most people are asymptomatic, about half get flu-like illness, rash, sore throat and fever

Incubation period (time from infection to initial symptoms): 14 - 28 days (if initial symptoms do in fact appear)

Window period (time from infection to blood tests turning "positive"): 10-14 days (genetic tests) to 30-90 days (antibody tests)

Unaware they have HIV: 15–20 percent, especially in younger individuals and minorities

What happens if no treatment: 99 percent progress to debilitating immunosuppression leading to AIDS ten to twelve years after infection. Death comes two to three years after the onset of AIDS (AIDS equals new unexplained weight loss, fever, enlarged lymph nodes, rare infections and cancers)

Source of HIV infection: Blood, cum, pre-cum, rectal or vaginal secretions (increased risk with menstruation), breast milk

Infectivity (Risk of transmission after one condom-less sex act with untreated patient or HIV tainted blood):

Extreme: Blood transfusion: 93 percent risk transmission from HIV positive blood
Vaginal delivery: 25 percent risk from untreated HIV positive mother
Breast feeding: 10 percent risk from untreated HIV positive mother

High: Anal sex, receptive/bottom: 1.4 percent risk from untreated HIV positive partner
Needle sharing/drug use: 0.7 percent risk from untreated HIV positive partner

Moderate: Anal sex: Insertive (top): 0.1 percent risk from untreated HIV positive partner
Needle stick (accident): 0.23 percent risk from untreated HIV positive source

Low: Vaginal sex, infected male: 0.08 percent risk (4 percent/year if weekly sex)
Vaginal sex, infected female: 0.04 percent risk (2 percent/year if weekly sex)

Negligible: Receptive oral sex (5 documented cases), blood transfusion in U.S. (0.00004 percent), sharing sex toys (one case)

Zero: Kissing, household contacts (showers, toilet seats, towels), saliva, tears, hugs, shaking hands, shared personal objects, food or water

Things that change infectivity: In the first several months after HIV infection, viral load skyrockets, increasing infectiousness by as much as 26-fold. So, during that time, the per-sex-act risk of receptive vaginal transmission jumps from 0.08 percent to 2 percent; the risk of one episode of receptive anal sex goes from 1.4 percent to 33 percent!

Curable?   No

Treatable? Yes; Anti-retroviral treatment (ART)

Prevention (percent risk reduction):
1. Testing, especially for those at highest risk
2. Mutual monogamy with uninfected partner (100)
3. Optimal anti-retroviral therapy by HIV-infected persons (99 – 100)
4. Optimal pre-exposure prophylaxis (PrEP) use before high risk sex (99 plus)
5. Optimal post exposure prophylaxis (PEP) (28-day medication regimen taken after unprotected high risk sex) (95 plus)
6. Condoms (80)
7. Circumcision (65)
8. Detection and treatment of another co-existing STD

2. Quickie HPV Overview (Chapter 7)

Human papilloma virus (HPV) has recently emerged from the shadow of HIV as Americas deadliest STD - HPV associated cancers now kill twice as many Americans (13,000) as HIV (6,700). HPV is 80 – 90 percent preventable with Gardasil 9 vaccination, but no anti-HPV treatment exists.

Without vaccination, essentially every sexually active individual will catch one or more of the 37 strains of HPV – 5 percent of persons will get visible oral or genital warts, 1 percent will get invasive rectal, penile, cervical, vaginal or oral cancers. 90 percent of infected individuals silently clear the virus within the first few years – so unless an abnormal PAP or screening HPV test is found, the vast majority remain totally unaware of their HPV infection.

HPV is readily passed skin to skin. Hair removal can damage the integrity of the skin for several days and markedly increase the chance of HPV infection. Although condoms prevent transmission to or from the covered penis, open territory exists, thus the chance of HPV transmission is only lowered by 50 percent.

Current and formerly sexually active women must screen for HPV associated rectal, vaginal, vulvar and cervical cancers (a pelvic examination together with a PAP smear every three years from age 21 to 30 then switch to an every 5-year HPV test until age 65). Men must stay on alert for HPV associated oral cancer (MSM for oral and anal cancer) but no cancer prevention strategy has been validated yet - although screening for high risk HPV strains makes logical sense.

Bottom line, if you are having sex — with or without a condom — make sure you are vaccinated against HPV, if appropriate. The younger and less sexually experienced an individual is, the more effective the vaccine. The vaccine is FDA-approved (in other words your health insurance will reimburse you for cost) up until age 45.

HPV Summary:

Incidence (new U.S. cases/yr.):   14,000,000

Prevalence (total U.S. cases):   79,000,000

Initial symptoms: Majority of people are asymptomatic

Incubation period (time from infection to illness): 90 days for warts, 10 - 30 years for cancers

Window period (time from infection to blood tests turning "positive"): 90 days (genetic tests)

What happens if no treatment (i.e. prevention): 10 percent of infected individual will not be able to clear the virus over the first several years (a persistent infection). 5 percent of those with a persistent high-risk strain will eventually develop cervical, vaginal, penile, anal or oro-pharyngeal cancer. Some skin, esophageal and lung cancer might also be HPV related.

5 percent of those infected with a low risk strain will develop visible oral or genital warts.

Source of infection: Skin to skin contact via vaginal, rectal or oral sex or touching

Infectivity (Risk of transmission after one condom-less sex act with untreated patient):

Extreme: Sex toys

High: Anal sex: infected male penis to anus (1 percent), fellatio, cunnilingus, romantic touching (petting, hand job, fingering)

Moderate: Vaginal sex: Infected male (0.4 percent)

                                 Infected female (0.4 percent)

              French kissing

Negligible: Toilet seats, gym machines, damp towels

Zero: Blood, breast feeding, tears, swimming pools or hot tubs, hugs, shaking hands, shared personal hygiene objects, food or water

Things that change infectivity: Extreme pubic grooming within several days of sexual contact may increase HPV infectivity 4-fold

Test (accuracy): High risk HPV testing (95 – 99 percent), PAP (95 percent)

Curable? No

Treatable? No current anti-viral HPV medication but warts may be treated as well as precancerous lesions

Prevention (percent risk reduction if known):

1. Vaccination for the 9 strains (Gardasil-9) that cause most warts and cancers ideally at ages 11-12 but approved until age 45 (99 for persistent HPV infection)
2. Condoms (50)
3. HPV testing (cervix) every 5 years beginning age 30 until age 65 (95-99)
4. PAP smear every 3 years age 21 to 30 (95)
5. HPV testing of other tissues (anal, vulvar, penile, oral or esophageal) makes logical sense but is still of unproven value for cancer prevention
6. Circumcision
7. Avoid sex within 48 hrs of skin shaving
8. Avoid sex during active STD, including herpes
9. Treat visible vaginal warts pre-vaginal delivery (may decrease respiratory papillomatosis in newborn)
10. Stop tobacco smoking
11. Ideal health (fitness, weight and sleep) to aid the body's immune system

3. Quickie Hepatitis B Overview (Chapter 9)

Hepatitis B is similar to HIV in that it's passed via oral, vaginal or anal sex, childbirth, tainted blood products or shared needles among intravenous drug users. But Hepatitis B is tenfold more infectious than HIV. And Hepatitis B is totally preventable - Hepatitis B vaccination is 99 percent effective and safe. Hepatitis B is a universal infant vaccine. Since 1991 almost all newborns in the United States have been vaccinated.

Hepatitis B infects liver cells of unimmunized individuals, sometimes with no symptoms, sometimes causing a severe illness with extreme exhaustion, jaundice (yellowing of eyes and skin) and itchiness. Hepatitis B is then either naturally vanquished by the body's immune system (95 percent of the time in adults but only 10 percent of time in infants) or it persists for life, resulting decades later in liver damage, cirrhosis, liver cancer and early death.

Hepatitis B infections have been dramatically reduced since the1991 introduction of the extremely effective Hepatitis B vaccination. People from countries not requiring infant vaccination, however, means hundreds of thousands of Americans (422,000) still live with persistent Hepatitis B infection (mostly asymptomatic). There is no cure for those individuals, but recently, excellent treatments —lifelong anti-Hepatitis B medicines similar to the lifelong anti-viral treatments needed to control HIV — have been discovered.

Bottom line, everyone without a prior vaccine history should get a one-time Hepatitis B test — and if unprotected, the Hepatitis B vaccine.

Hepatitis B Summary:

Incidence (new U.S. cases/year):   19,000

Prevalence (total U.S. cases):   420,000

Initial symptoms: Majority of acute adult infections are asymptomatic but acute Hepatitis B infection, ranging from a mild illness with few or no symptoms to a serious condition requiring hospitalization, can cause exhaustion, jaundice (yellowing of eyes and skin) and itchiness

Incubation period (time from infection to initial symptoms): 60 to 90 days

Window period (time from infection to blood tests turning "positive"): 30 to 60 days (antibody tests)

What happens if no treatment: A new adult infection results in exhaustion, jaundice (yellowing of eyes and skin) and itchiness; 5 percent go on to cirrhosis, liver cancer and need liver transplantation

Source of infection: Oral, vaginal or anal sex (increased risk with ejaculation), childbirth or tainted Hepatitis B blood products or shared needles among intravenous drug users

Infectivity (Risk of transmission after one condom-less sex act with untreated patient):

    High: Shared needles among intravenous IV drug users

    Moderate: Anal sex   from infected male – 12 percent risk transmission
               Vaginal sex: From infected male – 0.7 percent risk transmission
               From infected female - 0.35 percent risk transmission

Low: Oral sex, French kissing, sex toys

Zero: Breast feeding, coughing or sneezing, tears, hugs, shaking hands, shared personal objects, food or water

Things that change infectivity: More readily spread with ejaculation

Test (accuracy): Hepatitis B antibody blood test, DNA confirmatory blood test (99 percent)

Curable? No

Treatable? Yes, lifelong anti-Hepatitis B medicines (similar to the lifelong anti-viral treatments needed to control HIV)

Prevention (percent risk reduction if known):
1. Vaccination (99)
2. Condoms (80)
3. Mutual monogamy with uninfected (based on screening blood test(s)) partner (100)
4. One-time Hepatitis B test for unvaccinated individuals or persons born in high risk part of the world

4. Quickie Hepatitis C Overview (Chapter 9)

Hepatitis C is the most lethal viral hepatitis. Half of Hepatitis C infections lead to persistent life-long asymptomatic infections – about 30 percent will then, decades later, progress to cirrhosis, liver cancer and early death.

Hepatitis C, like Hepatitis A and Hepatitis B, primarily infects liver cells. It also sometimes presents with no obvious symptoms but often can cause a severe illness with extreme exhaustion, jaundice and itchiness. The lack of an effective vaccination means compared to Hepatitis B, Hepatitis C is much more common – fully 3,500,000 Americans have it, many of whom were born between 1945 and 1964, the "baby boomer" generation. Today, new Hepatitis C infections mainly occur among IV drug users who share needles and in some MSM who engage in high risk sexual activity. Hepatitis C is 20-fold less contagious than Hepatitis B with vaginal sex and thus only infrequently transmitted during vaginal sex or childbirth. In the 1950's and 60's, many Americans unknowingly contracted Hepatitis C, perhaps by some hygiene lapse (possibly by reuse of needles or non-sterile equipment) at doctors' offices, clinics or hospitals.

Hepatitis C is the one viral STD with a complete cure! Since 2014, three separate hepatitis C antiviral cures have been released (successful treatment lengths vary from 8 to 12 weeks). There is currently no preventative vaccine for Hepatitis C. Condoms may help in high risk populations, but as mentioned above, sexual transmission is very uncommon.

Bottom line, a cure is available so it's important we screen all individuals for occult Hepatitis C - everyone should take a one-time Hep C blood test, especially individuals born in the 1950s or 60s. Intravenous drug users and MSM with ongoing risks of contracting Hepatitis C need a yearly blood test.

Hepatitis C Summary:

Incidence (new U.S. cases/year):   31,000

Prevalence (total U.S. cases):   3,500,000 (2 percent of those born in the 50s and 60s)

Initial symptoms: Majority of people are asymptomatic

Incubation period (time from infection to illness): 60 days to years

Window period (time from infection to blood tests turning "positive"): 30 to 60 days (antibody tests)

What happens if no treatment: Acute adult infection results in exhaustion, jaundice and itchiness; 50 percent spontaneously heal, 50 percent go on to persistent lifelong infection, 30 percent of the persistently infected individuals get cirrhosis, liver cancer and need liver transplantation

Source of infection: Contaminated blood products, "dirty" needles for drug use or medical use, possible sharing of drug use equipment, rarely sex or childbirth

Infectivity: (Risk of transmission after one condom-less sex act with untreated patient):
  High: Shared needles by intravenous drug users
  Low: Anal sex with trauma, blood - 0.05 percent risk transmission (2 percent/year with weekly sex)
        Vaginal sex: Infected male - 0.025 percent risk transmission (1 percent/year with weekly sex)

Infected female - 0.02 percent risk transmission (1 percent/year with   weekly sex)
Childbirth

Negligible: Sex toys, oral sex, French kissing

Zero: Breast feeding, tears, hugs, shaking hands, shared personal objects, food or water

Test (accuracy): Hepatitis C antibody blood test, DNA confirmatory blood test (99 percent)

Curable?   Nearly 100% as of 2014!

Treatable? Yes! Various once-a-day hepatitis C antiviral therapies for 8 - 12 weeks.

Prevention (percent risk reduction):
1. Condoms (80)
2. Mutual monogamy with uninfected (based on screening blood test(s)) partner (100)
3. One-time Hepatitis C blood test for everyone
4. Yearly screening for those at risk (intravenous drug users and some MSM)

5. Quickie Herpes Simplex Virus Type 1 and 2 (HSV1 and HSV2) Overview (Chapter 11)

Four decades ago, HSV was no big deal. The rash was transient. The symptoms were mild or nonexistent. Sometimes "cold" sores popped out on the edge of the lip (HSV1). Sometimes the "cold" sores appeared on the genitals (HSV2). Who cared?

Then Americans panicked. The media and big pharma exaggerated tales of the "bad" genital herpes (HSV2): recurrent attacks (in truth rare), extremely painful attacks (in truth rare), childbirth disasters (in truth extremely rare), contagiousness (in truth minimal, i.e. only 1 transmission per one to two thousand sexual exposures) and incurability (true, but so what?). The biggest misconception? HSV2 is the genital, bad herpes. In truth, HSV1 is now the cause of over half of all genital herpes infections.

Both HSV1 and HSV2 infections are typically symptom free. HSV2 essentially only infects genital regions. HSV1 can infect either oral or genital regions. When symptomatic, genital HSV1 presents with small clusters of genital blisters, indistinguishable from HSV2. Both outbreaks look exactly the same. Both outbreaks shed virus when lesions are present. Both outbreaks can shed virus silently about 3 days a month (when no lesions can be seen). In terms of the very rare chance of spread during childbirth, HSV1 is equal if not more of a threat than HSV2.

In America, the frequency of HSV2 is declining – in 2010 16 percent had HSV2 compared with 12 percent in 2016 of adults aged 16-49. Women are twice as likely as men to be infected with HSV2 because of anatomic differences that make it easier for the female genitalia to get infected. HSV1 is also declining - 58 percent (2010) compared with 48 percent (2018) of adults aged 16-49. Eighty percent of Americans older than 70 have HSV1. Women have 20 percent more HSV1 infections than men.

It's possible to get genital herpes merely by rubbing your skin in the "boxer shorts" regions — or having oral contact — with the "boxer shorts" skin of someone actively shedding herpes virus. You can get genital HSV2 or genital HSV1 from a partner who has absolutely never had symptoms or any visible skin findings. Those individuals unaware they are HSV positive transmit the vast majority of new adult genital herpes infections

If you don't have herpes: test! Many mistakenly believe they don't have herpes based on never having suspicious symptoms and their doctor never running an accurate herpes test. Also test your partners. Remember it takes 4 weeks for the usual herpes tests to turn positive. Keep your skin barrier intact. Avoid pubic grooming two days prior to sexual contact. Use condoms always (50 percent reduced risk). Lastly, consider this unproven but scientifically plausible approach: Pre-exposure prophylaxis with valacyclovir (or acyclovir) before sex.

If you know you have genital herpes: Tell your partner (50 percent reduced risk), always use condoms (50 percent reduced risk) and go on daily valacyclovir or acyclovir (50 percent reduced risk) and lastly avoid pubic grooming in the several days prior to sex.

Bottom line, herpes stigma is unwarranted. The HSV1 strain is not exactly "good," on the other hand, the HSV2 strain is really not so "bad."

HSV-2 Summary:

Incidence (new U.S. cases/year):   1,400,000 (essentially all genital)

Prevalence (total U.S. cases):   30,000,000

Initial symptoms: Majority of people are asymptomatic. Occasionally, HSV2 presents with groups of small blisters/irritations over the genital, buttock or low back regions

Rarely (< 1 percent) new infections may show up as headache, stiff neck and high fever similar to meningitis.

Incubation period (time from infection to illness): 3 - 12 days for symptoms to appear (if they do appear)

Window period (time from infection to blood tests turning "positive"): 14 days (genetic tests) 30 to 45 days (antibody tests)

What happens if no treatment: Recurrent noticeable sores/irritations (10 percent) (about 3 - 4 times per year)

Severe recurrent attacks (< 1 percent) possibly including headaches, stiff neck and total body "flu" complaints

Infection of newborn during vaginal child birth rare (< 0.02 percent), but very serious

Source of infection:
  a) If recurrent obvious symptoms (10 percent): Virus sheds a day prior and during outbreaks and also sheds silently in-between outbreaks
  b) If recurrent minor, or unidentified symptoms (40 percent): Virus sheds just before and during outbreaks and also sheds silently in-between outbreaks
  c) If no symptoms (50 percent): Virus sheds intermittently (about 3 days a month) thru genital/anal skin

Infectivity (Risk of transmission after *one* condom-less sex act with untreated patient):

Moderate: Vaginal sex, from infected male – 0.1 percent risk transmission (5 percent a year)
Vaginal sex, from infected female - 0.05 percent risk transmission (3 percent a year)
Anal sex

Low: Sex toys, vaginal delivery, romantic touching (petting, hand job)

Negligible: Oral sex, French kissing

Zero: Breast feeding, tears, hugs, shaking hands, shared personal objects, food or water

Things that change infectivity: Extreme pubic grooming within several days of sexual contact may increase HSV infectivity 4-fold.

Test (accuracy): Two-stage: Herpes Select antibody PLUS confirmatory Western Blot antibody tests (95-99 percent) or swab DNA test taken from active lesion(s) (99 percent)

Curable? No

Treatable? Yes, various doses of valacyclovir, acyclovir or famciclovir 2 - 3 times a day for several days.

Prevention (percent risk reduction if known):
1. Condom (50)
2. HSV screening tests and if positive, partner notification (50)
3. Reduced transmission to others: Those infected take a daily antiviral drug (valacyclovir 500 to 1000 mg) (50)
4. Avoid sex during active symptomatic breakout (wait until sores fully heal)
5. Mutual monogamy with uninfected (based on accurate screening blood test) partner (100)
6. Avoid sex within 48 hrs of skin shaving
7. Test yourself (remember it takes on average 4 - 6 weeks for the usual herpes test to turn positive)
8. Test new partners
9. Make sure your doctor uses the accurate two-test-process to diagnose HSV2 infection
10. Pre-exposure prophylaxis with 500 to 1000 mg valacyclovir (unproven but possible)

HSV-1 Summary:

Incidence (new U.S. cases/year):   400,000 (oral, adult onset)
                                          1,200,000 (genital, adult onset)
                                          1,600,000 (oral, childhood onset)

Prevalence (total U.S. cases):   35,000,000 (oral, adult onset)
                                          25,000,000 (genital, adult onset)
                                          67,000,000 (oral, childhood onset)

Initial symptoms: Majority of people are asymptomatic. Occasionally, HSV1 presents with groups of small blisters or sores over either oral/facial or genital /buttock/low back regions

Incubation period (time from infection to illness): 3 - 12 days for symptoms to appear (if they do appear)

Window period (time from infection to blood tests turning "positive"): 14 days (genetic tests) 30 to 45 days (antibody tests)

What happens if no treatment: Recurrent noticeable sores/irritations (10 percent) (less frequent than HSV2)

Severe recurrent attacks (< 1 percent) possibly including headaches, stiff neck and total body "flu" complaints (less severe than HSV2)

Infection of newborn vaginal child birth rare (< 0.03 percent), but very serious

Source of infection: Individuals shedding HSV1 silently or via oral/facial, genital or anal sores

Infectivity (Risk of transmission after one condom-less sex act with untreated patient):

    Moderate: Vaginal sex, infected male – 0.1 percent risk transmission (5 percent year)
                     Vaginal sex, infected female - 0.05 percent risk transmission (3 percent year)
                     Oral Sex
    Low: Sex toys, vaginal delivery, French kissing, romantic touching (petting, hand job, fingering), kissing and sharing sex toys
    Zero: Breast feeding, tears, hugs, shaking hands, shared personal objects, food or water
    Test (accuracy): Two-stage Herpes Select antibody blood test (95 - 99 percent) with Western blot confirmation or swab HSV1 DNA test taken from active lesion(s) (99 percent) (blood tests can not differentiate between oral or genital infection)
    Curable?   No
    Treatable? Valacyclovir (antiviral) 2000 mg immediately at onset symptoms then repeat one time 12 hours later or other antivirals like acyclovir or famciclovir at different doses

Prevention (percent risk reduction):
    1. Condom (50)
    2. HSV screening tests and if positive, partner notification (50)
    3. Avoid sex during active symptomatic breakout (wait till lesions fully heal)
    4. Mutual monogamy with uninfected (based on accurate screening blood test) partner (100)
    5. Avoid sex within 48 hrs of skin shaving
    6. Pre-exposure prophylaxis with 500 to 1000 mg valacyclovir (unproven but possible)

6. Quickie Syphilis Overview (Chapter 12)

Syphilis, a deadly bacterial STD that can cannibalize the body from the inside, has reshaped human history - syphilis dementia has affected a veritable who's who of former world leaders. At its zenith, from the 1600's thru the early 1800's, one in five Europeans was infected. Finally, with the advent of antibiotics in the 1940's, syphilis was almost completely eradicated.

But now this corkscrew syphilis bacterium – 500-fold more infectious than HIV - is making an improbable comeback. 88,000 Americans got syphilis last year, a 300 percent increase over the last decade. But that's nothing compared to the situation in South East Asia and Sub Saharan Africa where 8 *million* new cases of this totally treatable malady occur yearly.

Syphilis manifests as superficial painless open sores with heaped-up edges (chancers) on genital skin or in the mouth two to twelve weeks after exposure. It transmits to others with skin to skin contact via kissing, oral, vaginal or anal sex or childbirth. This skin to skin spread (similar to HPV and HSV) lowers the protective effect of condoms to just 50 percent.

If syphilis lesions are ignored, they will entirely resolve. But don't think it's gone. Several months later, the syphilis bacteria reemerge in a second stage characterized by a measles like skin rash and/or sores in the mouth, vagina, or anus along with fever, swollen lymph nodes, and body aches. Those symptoms also completely resolve without treatment. Then, Katie bar the door! Stage three can present months to years later: catastrophic eye, heart, blood vessel, and or brain damage, i.e. the frontpage disaster being progressive dementia.

Syphilis can be easily and accurately diagnosed with a VDRL or RPR screening blood test and if positive (10 - 90 days after exposure) a confirmatory treponemal antibody test is needed.

Unlike the vast majority of viral STDs, all bacterial STDs are completely curable with antibiotics. Penicillin fully cures syphilis, but if treatment begins in the late stages, some organs may have irreversible damage. The route and amount of penicillin depends on the duration of the disease.

Condoms are helpful (50 percent protection) but not a panacea. Testing is key, especially for those at highest risk: heterosexuals with multiple partners should test yearly and MSM with multiple partners should test every 3 months. Avoid sex within 48 hrs of pubic hair removal. Pre-exposure prophylaxis with doxycycline is also effective for high risk individuals.

Bottom line, syphilis is readily curable. All pregnant women and those sexually active with multiple partners should get tested at least once a year.

Syphilis Summary:

Incidence (new U.S. cases/year):   88,000

Prevalence (total U.S. cases):   120,000 (few cases stay undiagnosed and persist into stage three)

Initial symptoms: Majority are asymptomatic. Sometimes a painless, firm, dime-sized lesion (chancre) appears anywhere on oral-genital skin

Incubation period (time from infection to illness): 10 to 90 days

What happens if no treatment: 1-3 months after the initial chancre (painless sore), a total body rash with symptoms of fever, tiredness and swollen glands may appear. 25 percent of infected individuals then progress over the next decade to permanent eye, heart and brain damage.

Source of infection: Skin to skin transmission from oral, vaginal and anal sex and less likely kissing, childbirth and rarely blood transfusions

Infectivity (Risk of transmission after one condom less sex act with untreated patient)

    High: Vaginal sex, infected male – 30 percent risk transmission
                    Vaginal sex, infected female – 30 percent risk transmission
                    Anal sex, infected male – 30 percent risk transmission
                    Oral sex, infected male – 30 percent risk transmission

    Moderate: French kissing

    Low: Kissing, sex toys, romantic touch (petting, hand job, fingering), childbirth

    Negligible: Blood transfusions (in U.S.)

    Not infectious: Breast feeding, tears, hugs, shaking hands, shared personal objects, food or water

    Test (accuracy): Syphilis antibody test, confirmed by treponemal test (99 percent)

    Curable? Yes, if detected in early stages

    Treatable? Yes, penicillin injections depending on duration of disease.
                  Primary or secondary syphilis or syphilis of less than one-year duration:
                  Penicillin injection, one dose. Treated people need to abstain from sexual contact for 7 days.

                  Syphilis of unknown duration with absolutely no signs or symptoms:
                  Penicillin injection, weekly for 3 weeks. Treated people need to abstain from sexual contact for 21 days.

                  Third stage disease, any evidence of eye, heart, or brain involvement:
                  Penicillin intravenous for 2 weeks, then a penicillin injection.

Prevention (percent risk reduction if known):

    1. Condoms (50)
    2. Mutual monogamy with uninfected (based on screening blood tests) partner (100)
    3. Testing, especially for those at highest risk: heterosexuals with multiple partners or in MSM with multiple partners every 3 months to one year
    4. Avoid sex within 48 hrs of skin shaving
    5. PrEP/PEP (pre- or post-exposure prophylaxis): 100 mg of doxycycline daily or 200 mg of doxycycline one time before or immediately after sex

7. Quickie Gonorrhea Overview (Chapter 14)

The old testament book of Leviticus describes gonorrheal "urethral discharge" and the associated disgust, shame, and perceived uncleanliness. Flash forward to today: The biblical description still holds true! And recent internet headlines show gonorrhea is still all too "relevant."
Gonorrhea Rates Jump 67percent in US, Reach Record High.
Drug-Resistant Super–Gonorrhea Is Here – That Means an Antibiotic Crisis Is Here Too.

You get gonorrhea when an infected source — vagina, penile, rectum, throat, saliva or occasionally fingers — contacts a mucous membrane lining. Australian studies show some men spread gonorrhea via deep kissing or saliva without any sexual contact.

Men are more likely to get gonorrhea symptoms than women. Men often get a scant penile drip which intensifies over 24 hours to obvious pus. In women, silent infections are common and especially dangerous as treatment is typically delayed. Some women notice a thin, purulent, mildly foul-smelling vaginal discharge with some pain on urination. Throat and anal infections are most often asymptomatic but can show up with throat aches or rectal itchiness, mucous discharge and the urge to defecate. If you have atypical urinary or vaginal symptoms, don't live in denial! 40 percent of men and 50 percent of woman with gonorrhea at an STD clinic reported continuing to have sex despite suspicious complaints. That is how the disease spreads. In addition, silent gonorrhea infections are dangerous because treatment is delayed for months before the disease either spontaneously resolves (80 percent) or progresses up the reproductive tract (20 percent) to inflame, scar and permanently damage Fallopian tubes and internal reproductive organs.

Test for gonorrhea with accurate urine (or if appropriate throat, vagina, or rectal swabs) DNA assays that are positive within days of exposure. There is still a 100 percent cure rate but as noted above, antibiotic resistance has begun to emerge. Avoid sex for seven days after treatment. Inform all sex contacts and kissing partners from the last 60 days. Meningococcal B vaccination appears to be protective against future gonorrhea. Urinating after sex may also decrease infection (up to 30 percent effective). Condoms are also very helpful (80 percent effective).

Bottom line, get tested. Gonorrhea is curable.   If you are sexually active, get regular screening tests to detect occult disease and prevent serious long-term reproductive complications.

Gonorrhea Summary:

Incidence (new U.S. cases/year):   820,000

Prevalence (total U.S. cases):   250,000 (The low number of total U.S. cases is because gonorrhea infection only lasts a few months - so there are more new cases (incidence) than the number of total cases (prevalence) at any single point in time.)

Initial symptoms: 50 percent of men present initially with abnormal penile discharge that intensifies over the ensuing 24 hours. Most women are asymptomatic but some report increasing vaginal discharge, pain on urination or pain with intercourse

Incubation period (time from infection to illness): 1-3 days

Window period (time from infection to blood tests turning "positive"): 1-2 days (genetic tests)

What happens if no treatment: Asymptomatic gonorrhea may go undetected for months before either spontaneously resolving (80 percent) or progressing up the reproductive tract (20 percent) to inflame, scar and permanently damage Fallopian tubes and internal reproductive organs

Source of infection: Infected saliva, throat, vaginal, penile and rectal secretions. There is increased risk with ejaculation and with menstruation

Infectivity (Risk of transmission after one condom-less sex act with untreated patient):

Very High: Vaginal sex from infected male – 60 percent risk transmission
Vaginal sex from infected female – 25 percent risk transmission
Anal sex from infected male – 80 - 90 percent risk transmission
Oral sex from infected male – 60 - 70 percent risk transmission

High: French kissing and use of saliva as sexual lubricant

Moderate: Sex toys

Low: Romantic touching (petting, hand job, fingering)

Negligible: Towels, especially damp; household transmission rare

Zero: Breast feeding, tears, hugs, shaking hands, food or water

Test (accuracy): DNA urine or vaginal/throat/rectal swab test (99 percent)

Curable? 100 percent

Treatment? Ceftriaxone 250 intramuscular injection plus azithromycin 1 gram orally

Prevention (percent risk reduction if known):
1. Testing, especially for those at highest risk (young women and MSM)
2. Mutual monogamy with uninfected (based on screening tests) partner (100)
3. Condom (80)
4. Meningococcal B vaccination (30)
5. Be alert for clues of atypical gonorrhea: Discharge, urinary discomfort, between cycle bleeding, heavy periods, pain with intercourse or joint/skin problems
6. STDs often travel in pairs! If you have a new case of chlamydia, Trich or HSV, don't forget to test for gonorrhea and HIV

8. Quickie Chlamydia Overview (Chapter 15)

Chlamydial is the gorilla in the room. At this very moment, nearly 3 million Americans are living with this STD – for many, infertility is the price to be paid.

Chlamydia is very common (4 times more common than gonorrhea). It's especially common in women under 25 - an immature cervix may be more susceptible to infection. It's very infectious — 650-fold more than HIV — via vaginal, oral, and rectal sex. It's hard to self-diagnose (70 percent of women and 50 percent of men with infections have no recognizable pelvic symptoms). Chlamydia is more dangerous than gonorrhea - occult chlamydia reproductive tract infections result in more scarring and complications than the more aggressive, symptomatic gonorrhea.

Thankfully, chlamydia is often a self-limiting disease: 80 percent spontaneously burn out and resolve after a year. However, up to 20 percent of the time, chlamydia scars uterine, tubal, and intra-abdominal surfaces, sometimes to the point of blocking the passage of a fertilized egg from the ovary to uterus implantation resulting in a life-threatening tubal pregnancy.

Whereas self-diagnosis is often near impossible, a screening urine (or if exposure dictates, a vaginal, anal or throat swab) DNA test is simple – and extremely accurate!

Antibiotic treatment is simple and 100 percent effective. The law now permits doctors to also give their patients extra antibiotic treatment for all recent at-risk partners. If your doctor is not offering this "expedited partner treatment", ask. It may be time to educate him or her!

Prevention includes mutual monogamy with uninfected (based on screening tests) partner (100 percent effective) condoms (80 percent effective) and pre-exposure treatment with daily doxycycline or post-exposure one time immediately after sex.

Bottom line, lack of symptoms is a curse; 130 *million* people worldwide wouldn't be blithely walking around with this infection if it were easy to self-diagnose! Be proactive. If you are sexually active — especially if you are a woman under 25 — get a yearly chlamydia test.

Chlamydia Summary:

Incidence (new U.S. cases/year): 2,900,000

Prevalence (total U.S. cases):   1,800,000 (If you are math oriented, the connection between incidence and prevalence is Prevalence = Incidence x Duration. When duration is less than 1 year, the prevalence will be less than the incidence. In this specific case, the duration for chlamydia is 4-6 months.)

Initial symptoms: Most cases are asymptomatic. 30 percent of women will have vaginal discharge or abnormal vaginal bleeding. Men may report scant thin penile discharge and or discomfort with urination

Incubation period (time from infection to illness): 1 to 4 weeks if symptoms do appear

Window period (time from infection to blood tests turning "positive"): 5 days (genetic tests)

What happens if no treatment: Many infections clear without consequence; however, 10 - 20

percent persist, proceeding to permanently damage pelvic organs leading to chronic pain or infertility. Chlamydia increases risk of contracting HIV 5-fold. It may rarely cause arthritis or even ovarian cancer.

Source of infection: Oral, vaginal, rectal (increased risk with ejaculation) sex or childbirth

Infectivity (Risk of transmission after one condom-less sex act with untreated patient):

High:	Vaginal sex from infected male – 50 percent risk transmission
	Vaginal sex from infected female –50 percent risk transmission
	Anal sex
Moderate:	Oral sex
Low:	French kissing, sex toys
Zero:	Breast feeding, tears, hugs, shaking hands, shared personal objects, food or water

Test (accuracy): DNA urine or vaginal/throat/rectal swab test (98 - 99 percent)

Curable?   Yes

Treatment? Yes: Azithromycin 1 gram, one oral dose or Doxycycline 100 mg, twice a day for 7 days

Prevention (percent risk reduction if known):

1. Condoms (80)
2. Mutual monogamy with uninfected (based on screening tests) partner (100)
3. PrEP/PEP (pre- or post-exposure prophylaxis): 100 mg of doxycycline daily or 200 mg of doxycycline one time before or immediately after sex

9. Quickie Mycoplasma Overview (Chapter 16)

Mycoplasma is brand new to the top ten STD list. It's been an STD suspect for years, but tests were too insensitive to convict it. Just now, a new accurate DNA test has changed all of that. Researchers now realize this very infectious (560-times more contagious than HIV) STD was causing millions of silent (70 percent) or minimally symptomatic (30 percent) chlamydia-like urethral, testicular, cervical, and fallopian tube infections. To complicate matters, mycoplasma is often resistant to the antibiotics used for chlamydia, gonorrhea, or trichomonas. So symptomatic or not, in many instances mycoplasma stays in the genital tract undiagnosed and often inappropriately treated with antibiotics aimed at chlamydia, poised to inflame the urethra, cervix, or fallopian tubes, contributing to America's infertility problem. In America today, one in nine young couples are infertile! Spoiler alert: a real-life *Handmaid's Tale*?

There are no good studies yet, but mycoplasma appears to be as common as chlamydia, so our best estimates are about 2.8 million new cases of mycoplasma in the U.S. each year. You get mycoplasma by exposure during condom-less sex to infected penile, vaginal, or rectal secretions. Best case, untreated mycoplasma remains silent and after an uneventful year the infection burns out. On the other hand, mycoplasma can form cause painful inflammation and permanent scarring inside genital structures. Mycoplasma also scars the fallopian tubes and may cause tubal pregnancy when the fertilized egg cannot make it through the blocked passageway from the ovaries into the uterus. There are about 1,000 maternal deaths yearly in the U.S. About 15 percent (150 deaths) of those deaths are due to tubal pregnancies. On that basis, every year mycoplasma, chlamydia, and gonorrhea are each responsible for up to 50 deaths.

One of the unique current challenges in the treatment of STDs: Doctors typically do not test for mycoplasma – they're unaware of a new DNA urine, vaginal or anal swab test that just became available in 2016 that can identify this treatable cause of infertility. Mycoplasma treatment is tricky because antibiotics ordinarily given for gonorrhea, chlamydia and Trich (other common STD causes of vaginal discharge) are not especially effective.

Condoms work to prevent infection, but they must be used correctly.

Bottom line, mycoplasma is a newly discovered STD. Be pro-active and ask about mycoplasma and and make sure you are being screened with the correct diagnostic test.

PS, blame me if the doctor gives you attitude!

Mycoplasma Summary:

Incidence (new U.S. cases/yr.):   2,800,000

Prevalence (total U.S. cases):   1,700,000

Initial symptoms: The majority of people are asymptomatic. 30 percent get symptoms: males may complain of thin, slightly milky penile (or rectal) discharge. Females may have unusual vaginal discharge, pain with sex or vaginal bleeding.

What happens if no treatment: Similar to chlamydia – long term pelvic pain and infertility

Incubation period (time from infection to illness): 7 to 28 days if symptoms do appear

Window period (time from infection to tests turning "positive"): 2-5 days (genetic tests)

Incubation Period: 7 - 14 days

Source of infection: Oral, vaginal, penile or rectal secretions (an increased risk with ejaculation)

Infectivity (Risk of transmission after one condom-less sex act with untreated patient):

High: Vaginal sex from infected male – 40-50 percent risk transmission
Vaginal sex from infected female – 30-40 percent risk transmission
Anal sex

Moderate: Oral sex

Mild: French kissing, sex toys

Zero: Breast feeding, tears, hugs, shaking hands, shared personal objects, food or water

Test (accuracy): DNA urine or vaginal/throat/rectal swab test (98 - 99 percent)

Curable? Yes

Treatable (percent success)? Yes; Moxifloxacin 400 mg by mouth for 10 days (70 – 100) or Azithromycin 1.5 - 2.5 gram by mouth one time (40 - 85) or Doxycycline 100 mg twice daily for 7 days followed by Azithromycin 1.5 gram over 2 days (>90)

Prevention (percent risk reduction if known):
1. Testing, especially for those at highest risk
2. Be proactive – ask about the new mycoplasma diagnostic test - most doctors still don't include it in their "thorough" STD panels
3. Condoms (80)
4. Mutual monogamy with uninfected (based on screening test) partner (100)

10. Quickie Trichomonas Overview (Chapter 17)

Almost 4 million Americans are currently living with an active parasitic STD - Trichomonas vaginalis - contracted through vaginal sex. It's very infectious - a 40 percent catch rate with a single episode of condom-less sex. It can cause minor urinary irritation or penile or vaginal discharge. It can cause vaginal malodor. But most of the time (85 percent), it causes no symptoms and people carry it without knowing it.

"Trich" triples the risk of acquiring HIV. It increases baby mortality (3 percent of pregnant women have Trich). Trich doesn't scar up reproductive tubes (like gonorrhea, chlamydia or mycoplasma) and typically spontaneously resolves but can also persist for years.

Trich is easy to diagnose with a urine or vaginal swab DNA test (95 percent accurate).

Trich is also easy to treat with antibiotics. However, twenty percent of folks treated for trichomoniasis get reinfected within three months, so like with every other STD, please tell all recent (within the last 60 days) contacts to get treated. Condoms are 80 percent effective in preventing transmission.

Bottom line, Trich is a curable parasite that can cause irritating symptoms and rarely complications during pregnancy.

Trichomonas Summary:

Incidence (new U.S. cases/yr.):   1,100,000

Prevalence (total U.S. cases):   3,700,000

Initial symptoms: 85 percent are asymptomatic. Symptomatic men can get minor urinary symptoms or a thin penile discharge. Women can report minimal urinary discomfort or a thin vaginal discharge, yellow to green, and occasionally foul smelling

Incubation period (time from infection to illness): 5 to 28 days (if symptoms do appear)

Window period (time from infection to blood tests turning "positive"): 2-5 days (genetic tests)

Incubation Period: 5 - 28 days

What happens if no treatment: Even asymptomatic trichomonas infection can increase one's risk of contracting HIV or cause pregnancy complications like preterm delivery.

Source of infection: Vaginal, penile and anal secretions (increased risk with ejaculation)

Infectivity (Risk of transmission after one condom-less sex act with untreated patient):
    High: Sex toys
    Moderate: Vaginal/anal sex infectivity is unknown, but presumed at least moderate
    Negligible: Oral sex, French kissing, romantic touching (petting, hand job, fingering), shared towels
    Zero: Breast feeding, tears, hugs, shaking hands, shared personal objects, food or water
    Test (accuracy): DNA urine or vaginal/rectal swab test (98 - 99 percent)
    Curable?   Yes
    Treatable? Yes; Metronidazole, 500 mg twice daily for 7 days
Prevention (percent risk reduction if known):
    1. Testing, especially for those at highest risk
    2. Condom effectiveness (80)
    3. Mutual monogamy with uninfected (based on screening test) partner (100)

11. Quickie Crabs (Pubic Lice) Overview (Chapter 18)

Pubic lice or "crabs" are different in three key ways from every other STD:

#1 You can see this STD – the pubic lice (nits) and its eggs are visible to the naked eye.

#2 There are relatively few silent infections; Pubic crabs almost always cause an obvious symptom – itchiness.

#3 Pubic lice are the dinosaurs of STDs. From approximately 3 million new pubic lice infestations each year in the 1990's, there has been an unprecedented 95 plus percent drop. The near global adaptation of pubic hair removal techniques, especially the "Brazilian," may be pushing pubic lice — which require pubic hair to survive — near extinction.

Public lice are spread to pubic hair via sexual contact. In rare instances, the infestation begins after contact with toilet seats, clothing, bed sheets and dirty towels used by an infected person.

Pubic itchiness begins approximately five to seven days after the initial pubic lice exposure. When skin is scratched hard enough, especially with long fingernails, bacterial boils or localized skin infection can result. Occasionally, the lice bites do not elicit an allergic response and itching never occurs. Rarely, individuals first see black residue (lice droppings) and miniscule white eggs in their underwear. Pubic lice do not spread any other disease or cause any internal medical complications.

The diagnosis of crabs is old-school: visual identification of lice (nits) and/or their eggs (with or without a magnifying glass).

Fortunately, effective treatment via creams or lotions (Nix, Rid) is available over the counter. The best prevention: Eliminate pubic hair. Condoms are of no benefit.

Bottom line, pubic lice — a nuisance parasite that carries no disease — is far less common now than just a decade ago. Nonetheless, if you have genital itchiness, look for the characteristic minute pubic crab and its eggs.

Pubic Lice Summary:

Incidence (new U.S. cases/yr.):   120,000

Prevalence (total U.S. cases):   60,000 (Pubic lice does not linger – almost always itchiness is present, meaning infected persons go for treatment promptly. Therefore, the new cases (incidence) is larger than the total cases at any one time (prevalence).)

Initial symptoms: Itchiness

What happens if no treatment: Itchiness leading to severe scratching that can result in bacterial streptococcal or staphylococcal infection of the skin

Incubation period (time from infection to illness): 7 to 14 days

Window period (time from infection to blood tests turning "positive"): 7 to 14 days (visual)

Source of infection: Vaginal or anal sex. Rarely, pubic lice can be contracted from contact with toilet seats, clothing, bed sheets or dirty towels used by an infected person

Infectivity (Risk of transmission after *one* condom-less sex act with untreated patient):

High: Vaginal sex (partners have pubic hair), romantic touching (petting, hand job, fingering)

Low: Oral sex, French kissing (eyebrows), shared personal objects

Negligible: Sex toys

Zero: Breast feeding, tears, hugs, shaking hands, food or water

Test (accuracy): Visual (unknown)

Curable? Yes

Treatable? Yes; 1 percent permethrin cream rinse or pyrethins with piperonyl butoxide (RID, Nix). Repeat treatment in 9–10 days if live lice are still found.

To kill any lice or nits remaining on clothing, towels, or bedding, machine-wash and machine-dry those items that the infested person used during the 2–3 days before treatment. Use hot water (at least 130°F) and the hot dryer cycle. Items that cannot be laundered can be dry-cleaned or stored in a sealed plastic bag for 2 weeks. All sex partners from within the previous month should be informed that they are at risk for infestation and should be treated. Persons should avoid sexual contact with their sex partner(s) until both they and their partners have been successfully treated and reevaluated to rule out persistent infestation.

Prevention (percent risk reduction if known):
1. Condoms are of no benefit in decreasing pubic crab infection
2. Complete pubic hair removal (100)

Non-Sexually Transmitted Genital Infection Capsule Summaries

Quickie Bacterial Vaginosis (BV) Overview (Chapter 19)

BV is the most common vaginal infection by a long shot – 30 percent of sexually active women have it – half with and half without obvious symptoms. BV is a sex-related but not sexually transmitted disease: It can start after a new partner. Condoms can prevent it. Non-sexually active women are rarely affected. However, there is no known male counterpart. Males get no symptoms and no disease. Furthermore, treating the male partner doesn't affect the women's chance of BV cure – or future recurrence.

BV symptoms include a milky thin vaginal discharge sometimes with a slightly fishy smell or merely vague vaginal discontent. There is overgrowth of Gardnerella or other unusual bacteria in the face of diminished levels of normal healthy vaginal bacteria like lactobacillus. BV is an imbalance of the normal bacterial in the vagina.

Women with BV are more likely to get other STDs, especially HIV, gonorrhea, chlamydia and herpes. They get more complications after abortions or other gynecological surgery. They get more pregnancy complications. A word of caution: It's tricky discerning normal vaginal discharge (which increases in pregnancy) and vaginal yeast overgrowth (also common during pregnancy) from BV discharge. Currently the detection and treatment of asymptomatic BV in pregnancy is controversial.

In the real-world, docs begin BV treatment if you have an adherent milky discharge with or without malodor and your urine DNA tests for gonorrhea, chlamydia, mycoplasma and Trich are all negative and you have no yeast discharge (it's usually a thicker "cottage cheese" consistency, but it can be thin, making it tough to differentiate from BV).

Very effective antibiotic pills or vaginal creams exist which also fortunately happen to be safe for pregnant women too. Treatment includes stopping tobacco. There is a two-to-three-fold increased chance of BV in cigarette smokers. Alcohol and bacterial vaginosis antibiotics don't mix, so avoid booze while on treatment.

Probiotic preparations or intravaginal non-medical lactobacillus (or yogurt) do not work. Triple sulfa intravaginal creams are not effective. Sex partners need not be notified or treated. Follow-up visits are unnecessary if symptoms resolve. Unfortunately, recurrent BV is common, so other empiric approaches — like switching to vaginal estrogen supplementation like the NuvaRing for birth control or monthly metronidazole treatment are occasionally required.

Bottom line, BV is very common and occasionally leads to post-operative and pregnancy complications. Don't be intimidated by health care providers who shoulder-shrug subtle discharge and odor complaints. Those docs erroneously believe BV symptoms are trivial and its diagnosis questionable. This pervasive misconception results in delayed and inadequate treatment.

Quickie Urinary Tract Infection Overview (Chapter 20)

UTI's are the most common genitourinary infection by a long shot – by age 24, a third of American women will have had at least one UTI heralded by discomfort in the act of urination, unnaturally frequent urination, an unnaturally urgent desire to urinate and occasionally blood in the urine.

First timers freak out, logically fearing they have contracted a raging STD. But UTIs are sex-related, not sexually transmitted. Intercourse tends to cause vaginal bacteria to migrate up to the urethra then into the sterile bladder – and urine is a pretty good bacterial culture medium, especially in pregnancy. UTIs appear about two days after intercourse, the time it takes for rapidly dividing bacteria to gain a foothold into the bladder wall. UTIs are so common after weddings that there's a special name for it: Honeymoon Cystitis.

Females get thirty-fold more UTIs than men because of anatomical differences: the distance from the tip of the urethra to the bladder is considerably longer in men (inches) compared with women (fractions of an inch). UTI's are not caused by sexually transmitted bacteria – males do not seem to be the source of UTIs in women. Condoms and spermicides do not lower UTI risk. Lastly, treatment of the male partner doesn't affect the women's chance of UTI cure – or future recurrence.

UTIs occasionally ascend up from the bladder via the ureter to cause kidney infection. That potentially dangerous complication that can lead to life threatening bloodstream infection is signaled by flank pain along the back, fever, chills, and general malaise.

UTI's are diagnosed by detecting white blood cells and abnormal numbers of bacteria in mid-stream urine collections. Antibiotic treatment is empiric ("an estimate") until culture results return. An over the counter urethral numbing agent can also be added to reduce urinary burning if it's severe – but just for the first few days. You don't want that numbing medicine on board at day three when the antibiotics should have markedly lowered or eliminated symptoms. Residual symptoms mean the antibiotic you are on may be ineffective and treatment changes should be considered. There is lots of conflicting information regarding cranberry products, most of it suggesting they do not work. Don't depend on them.

A urine culture returns in 48 - 72 hours. Assuming the correct antibiotic was originally given, no more than the three originally prescribed days of antibiotics is usually required. If the microbe is resistant to the initially prescribed antibiotic (less than 10 percent of the time), the appropriate drug is prescribed.

Being well hydrated is the best initial approach to preventing UTI's – it's safe, cost effective and scientifically validated! Merely consume an extra 1.5 liter per day - 2 extra cups of water three times a day to reduce recurrent UTI's by 50 percent.

Bottom line, UTIs are common, easily treatable with antibiotic and extra water but can be very uncomfortable. Do not "ride it out." If you think you have an UTI, get treated.

Quickie Yeast Overview (Chapter 21)

At any one time, up to half of all women have at least some vaginal yeast, but only 5 percent have any symptoms consistent with an "infection."

Eventually, over their life time, over three quarters of women will have a yeast "infection" with some or all of the following symptoms: itching at outer edge of the vagina, white "cottage cheese" discharge, outer vaginal discomfort with urination, vaginal soreness, swelling, redness, and pain with intercourse. Woman often self-treat with over-the-counter anti-fungal creams but self-diagnosis is an iffy proposition: Only half of those women actually have a yeast infection. The main "complication" of vaginal yeast infections is in fact incorrect self-diagnosis – delaying treatment of other more troublesome and serious causes of vaginal discharge, including BV, gonorrhea, chlamydia, mycoplasma or Trich.

Candidiasis is typically also a sex-related, not a sexually transmitted disease. Oral or vaginal sex can introduce yeast into the vagina. Elevated estrogen — occurring naturally in pregnancy and from birth control pills (BCPs) — increases risk. Up to 10 percent of male sex partners have yeast balanitis (often confused with herpes), characterized by red patchy areas on the glans of the penis and under the foreskin in conjunction with itching or irritation. Those men benefit from treatment with topical antifungal agents to relieve symptoms. Other than that, no partner treatment recommended. Frequent sexual activity and having multiple different partners does not increase the risk for vaginal yeast infections.

Diagnosis is based on the characteristic vaginal discharge plus yeast seen by microscopic exam or culture of a sample of the discharge.

Very effective anti-fungal treatment exists over the counter. Anti-fungal prescription pills are sometimes required. Some anti-fungal creams are oil-based and might weaken latex condoms. Acidophilus or probiotic treatments do not work and should be avoided.

Bottom line, yeast infections are common, cause few if any serious complications, and can be simply treated by over the counter medication. But if this home therapy is not promptly successful, seek medical help. Yeast is a true sexually transmitted disease in less than 10 percent of cases so mention it to your partner.

STD QUESTIONS AND ANSWERS

STD Statistics

1. TOP STDS- NEW INFECTIONS - EACH YEAR IN U.S.?

Sexually Transmitted Disease		New Infections each Year (U.S.)
Human Papilloma Virus (HPV)		14,000,000
All Herpes Simplex Virus (adult onset)		3,000,000
HSV1 – oral	400,000	
HSV1 - genital	1,200,000	
HSV2 - genital	1,400,000	
Chlamydia		2,900,000
Mycoplasma		2,800,000
Trichomonas		1,100,000
Gonorrhea		820,000
Pubic Lice		120,000
Syphilis		88,000
All Hepatitis		50,000
Hepatitis C Virus (Hep C)	31,000	
Hepatitis B Virus (Hep B)	19,000	
Human Immunodeficiency Virus (HIV)		38,400
TOTAL NEW STDS PER YEAR (U.S.)		**25 Million**
HSV1 oral, (childhood onset, not an STD)		**1,600,000**

2. TOP STDS- CURRENT INFECTIONS - EACH YEAR IN U.S.?

Sexually Transmitted Disease		Current Infections (U.S.)
Human Papilloma Virus (HPV)		79,000,000
All Genital Herpes Simplex Virus (adult onset)		55,000,000
HSV1 – oral	35,000,000	
HSV1 - genital (adult onset)	25,000,000	
HSV2 - genital	30,000,000	
Chlamydia		1,800,000
Mycoplasma		1,700,000
Trichomonas		3,700,000
Gonorrhea		250,000
Pubic Lice		120,000
Syphilis		120,000
All Hepatitis		3,920,000
(Hep C)	3,500,000	
(Hep B)	420,000	
Human Immunodeficiency Virus (HIV)		1,100,000
TOTAL CURRENT STDS CASES (U.S.)		**147 Million**
HSV1 oral, (childhood onset, not an STD)		**67,000,000**

3. TOP STDS - NEW INFECTIONS - EACH YEAR IN THE WORLD?

Sexually Transmitted Disease		New Infections Each Year (World)
Human Papilloma Virus (HPV)		unknown
All Herpes Simplex Virus (adult onset)		39,000,000
HSV1 – oral	8,000,000	
HSV1 - genital	8,000,000	
HSV2 - genital	23,000,000	
Chlamydia		130,000,000
Mycoplasma		unknown
Trichomonas		140,000,000
Gonorrhea		78,000,000
Pubic Lice		unknown
Syphilis		5,600,000
All Hepatitis		135,400,000
(Hep C)	5,400,000	
(Hep B)	135,400,000	
Human Immunodeficiency Virus (HIV)		1,800,000
TOTAL NEW STDs PER YEAR		**500 Plus Million**
HSV1 oral, (childhood onset, not an STD)		**102,000,000**

4. TOP STDS - CURRENT INFECTIONS - IN THE WORLD?

Sexually Transmitted Disease		Current Infections (World)
Human Papilloma Virus (HPV)		1,800,000,000
All Herpes Simplex Virus (adult onset)		830,000,000
HSV1 – oral	140,000,000	
HSV1 - genital	140,000,000	
HSV2 - genital	550,000,000	
Chlamydia		130,000,000
Mycoplasma		unknown
Trichomonas		100,000,000
Gonorrhea		27,000,000
Pubic Lice		unknown
Syphilis		18,000,000
All Hepatitis		400,000,000
(Hep C)	140,000,000	
(Hep B)	260,000,000	
Human Immunodeficiency Virus (HIV)		37,000,000
TOTAL NEW STDs PER YEAR		**3.3 Billion**
HSV1 oral, (childhood onset, not an STD)		**3,420,000,000**

5. HERPES SIMPLEX VIRUS 1 - CURRENT CASES - IN THE U.S?**

	2000	2010***	2016**
U. S. Population (millions)	281		323
Cases HSV1 (millions)	140		127
Childhood onset (not an STD)	72		67
All adult onset	66		60
oral	38		35
genital	28		25
Average (Ages 14 - 49) (%)	58	54	48
Ages 14 - 19 (%)	39	30	27
Ages 20 - 29 (%)	54	50	41
Ages 30 - 39 (%)	64	62	54
Ages 40 - 49 (%)	65	64	60
Ages > 70 (%)	90		
Male (%)			45
Female (%)			51
Non-Hispanic White (%)	52		37
Non-Hispanic Black (%)	68		59
Mexican-American (%)	82		72
Non-Hispanic Asian (%)	na		56

** NCHS Data Brief, No. 304, February 2018
***Bradley, H. Seroprevalence HSV1 and 2-U. S. 1999-2010.JID, Vol 209, Issue 3, Feb 1, 2014

6. HERPES SIMPLEX VIRUS 2 - NUMBER OF CURRENT CASES IN THE U.S. ?**

	2000	2010***	2016**
U. S. Population (millions)	281		323
Cases HSV2 (millions)	39		31
Ages 14 - 49 (%)	18	16	12
Ages 14 - 19 (%)	2	1	1
Ages 20 - 29 (%)	11	10	8
Ages 30 - 39 (%)	22	19	13
Ages 40 - 49 (%)	26	26	21
Male (%)	12	11	8
Female (%)	24	22	16
MSM (%)			22
Non-Hispanic White (%)	14		8
Non-Hispanic Black (%)	42		35
Mexican-American (%)	13		9
Non-Hispanic Asian (%)	na		4

** NCHS Data Brief, No. 304, February 2018
***Bradley, H. Seroprevalence HSV1 and 2-U. S. 1999 - 2010.JID, Vol 209, Issue 3, Feb 1, 2014

12 percent (percent of Americans between 14 and 49 with HSV2 in 2016) X 323 (U. S. population 2016 in millions) x 0.79 (percent of Americans over 16) = 31 million Americans with HSV2

^18 percent (percent of Americans between 14 and 49 with HSV2 in 2000) X 281 (U. S. population 2000 in millions) x 0.78 (percent of Americans over 16) = 39 million Americans with HSV2

STD Contagiousness

7. STD INFECTIVITY?

Top 10 STDs (U.S.)	Infectivity penis to vagina				Infectivity vagina to penis				Infectivity penis to throat				Infectivity penis to anus			
# exposures	1	3	10	52	1	3	10	52	1	3	10	52	1	3	10	52
HPV	0.40%	1%	4%	19%	0.40%	1%	4%	19%	unknown				1%	2%	6%	27%
HSV																
HSV1	0.1%	0.3%	1%	5%	0.05%	0.15%	0.5%	3%	unknown				unknown			
HSV2	0.1%	0.3%	1%	5%	0.05%	0.15%	0.5%	3%	unknown				unknown			
Chlamydia	50%	88%	100%	100%	25%	58%	94%	100%	unknown				unknown			
Mycoplasma	45%	83%	100%	100%	38%	76%	99%	100%	unknown				unknown			
Trichomonas	unknown				unknown				unknown				unknown			
Gonorrhea	60%	94%	100%	100%	25%	58%	94%	100%	63%	95%	100%	100%	84%	100%	100%	100%
Pubic Lice	unknown								unknown							
Syphilis	30%	66%	97%	100%	30%	66%	97%	100%	30%	66%	97%	100%	30%	66%	97%	100%
Hepatitis																
Hep C	0.025%	0.1%	0.2%	1%	0.02%	0.1%	0.2%	1%	negligible				unknown			
Hep B	0.7%	2%	7%	31%	0.35%	0.1%	3%	14%	negligible				12%	32%	72%	100%
HIV	0.08%	0.2%	1%	4%	0.04%	0.1%	0.4%	2%	negligible				1%	4%	13%	52%

$P = 100 \times (1-(1-z)^n)$

P= chance STD, z= infectivity, n= number of sexual exposures

8. CONDOM EFFECTIVENESS FOR STD PREVENTION?

Viral

HPV	50 percent
HSV1 – oral[2]	0 percent
HSV1 – genital[3]	50 percent
HSV2	50 percent
Hep C	80 percent
Hep B	80 percent
HIV	80 percent

Bacterial

Chlamydia	80 percent
Mycoplasma	80 percent
Gonorrhea	80 percent
Syphilis	50 percent

Parasitic

Trichomonas	80 percent
Pubic Lice	0 percent

[1]Assumes "typical use" of condoms
[2]Assumes rare use of condoms with oral sex
[3]Adult acquired

9. PERCENT OF AMERICA'S STDS PREVENTABLE WITH UNIVERSAL CONDOM USE?

Top 10 STDs		New Cases Each Year	Best Condom Effectiveness Prevent	Infections Universal Condom Use Could
Human Papilloma Virus (HPV)		14,000,000	50%	7,000,000
All Herpes Simplex Virus (HSV) (adult onset)		3,000,000		
HSV1 - oral		400,000	0%	0
HSV1 - genital		1,200,000	50%	600,000
HSV2 - genital		1,400,000	50%	700,000
Chlamydia		2,900,000	80%	2,320,000
Mycoplasma		2,800,000	80%	2,240,000
Trichomonas		1,100,000	80%	880,000
Gonorrhea		820,000	80%	656,000
Pubic Lice		120,000	0%	0
Syphilis		88,000	50%	44,000
All Hepatitis		50,000		
Hep C	31,000		80%	24,800
Hep B	19,100		80%	15,280
Human Immunodeficiency Virus	38,400		80%	30,720

Total Number New Cases each Year	**24,916,400**	
Number of new STD cases universal condom use could prevent		14,510,800
Percent of New STD Cases Condoms Could Prevent		**60 percent**

10. WHICH STDS TRANSMIT MUCH MORE WITH EJACULATION?

Viral
HPV	no
HSV1 – oral	no
HSV1 – genital	no
HSV2	no
Hep C	no
Hep B	**yes**
HIV	**yes**

Bacterial
Chlamydia	**yes**
Mycoplasma	**yes**
Gonorrhea	**yes**
Syphilis	no

Parasitic
Trichomonas	**yes**
Pubic Lice	no

11. DOES MENSTRUATION INCREASE THE CHANCE OF GETTING AN STD?

Viral
HPV	no
HSV1 – oral	no
HSV1 – genital	**possible increase**
HSV2	**possible increase**
Hep C	no
Hep B	no
HIV	**yes (for male and female partner)**

Bacterial
Chlamydia	**possible increase**
Mycoplasma	**possible increase**
Gonorrhea	**yes**
Syphilis	no

Parasitic
Trichomonas	no
Pubic Lice	no

12. WHICH STDS CAN YOU CATCH WITH ORAL SEX?

Viral
HPV   **very infectious**
HSV1 – oral^   **moderately infectious**
HSV1 – genital^   **moderately infectious**
HSV2   negligible infection risk
Hep C   negligible infection risk
Hep B   mildly infectious
HIV   negligible infection risk

Bacterial
Chlamydia   **moderately infectious**
Mycoplasma   **moderately infectious**
Gonorrhea   **extremely infectious**
Syphilis   **moderately infectious**

Parasitic
Trichomonas   negligible infection risk
Pubic Lice #   mildly infectious

^ Adult acquired
# Infection of eyebrows and eye lashes

13. HOW LIKELY IS FRENCH KISSING TO CAUSE STDS?

Viral
HPV   **moderately infectious**
HSV1 – oral   **mildly infectious**
HSV1 – genital   0
HSV2   negligible infection risk
Hep C   negligible infection risk
Hep B   mildly infectious
HIV   negligible infection risk (one case described)

Bacterial
Chlamydia   **mildly infectious**
Mycoplasma   **mildly infectious**
Gonorrhea   **very infectious**
Syphilis   **very infectious**

Parasitic
Trichomonas   negligible infection risk
Pubic Lice   negligible infection risk (eyebrows)

14. HOW LIKELY ARE SEX TOYS TO CAUSE STDS?

Viral
HPV	**extremely infectious**
HSV1 – oral	mildly infectious
HSV1– genital	mildly infectious
HSV2	mildly infectious
Hep C	negligible infection risk
Hep B	mildly infectious
HIV	negligible infection risk (one case documented)

Bacterial
Chlamydia	mildly infectious
Mycoplasma	mildly infectious
Gonorrhea	**moderately infectious**
Syphilis	mildly infectious

Parasitic
Trichomonas	**very infectious**
Pubic Lice	negligible infection risk

15. WHICH STDS CAN YOU CATCH WITH ROMANTIC TOUCHING (PETTING, HAND JOB, FINGERING)?

Viral
HPV	**very infectious**
HSV1 – oral	**mildly infectious**
HSV1 – genital	negligible infection risk
HSV2	0
Hep C	0
Hep B	0
HIV	0

Bacterial
Chlamydia	0
Mycoplasma	0
Gonorrhea	**mildly infectious**
Syphilis	**mildly infectious**

Parasitic
Trichomonas	**mildly infectious**
Pubic Lice	**very infectious**

16. ARE STDS PASSED NON-SEXUALLY – BY ROOMMATES, OR AIR BNB RENTERS IN BATHROOMS OR WOMEN TRYING ON CLOTHES IN DEPARTMENT STORES WITHOUT UNDERWEAR?

Viral
HPV	**rarely (bathroom floors for plantar warts (nonsexual))**
HSV1 – oral	negligible infection risk
HSV1 – genital	negligible infection risk
HSV2	negligible infection risk
Hep C	0
Hep B	0
HIV	0

Bacterial
Chlamydia	negligible infection risk
Mycoplasma	unknown
Gonorrhea	**rarely (moist towels, bedsheets or cloths)**
Syphilis	0

Parasitic
Trichomonas	**rarely (moist towels, bedsheets or cloths)**
Pubic Lice	**mildly infectious**

17. FOR EACH STD, WHAT IS THE MOST COMMON INITIAL PRESENTATION?

Viral
HPV	majority asymptomatic
HSV1 – oral	majority asymptomatic
HSV1 – genital	majority asymptomatic
HSV2	majority asymptomatic
Hep C	majority asymptomatic
Hep B	majority asymptomatic
HIV	majority asymptomatic

Bacterial
Chlamydia	majority asymptomatic
Mycoplasma	majority asymptomatic
Gonorrhea	majority asymptomatic (females)
	pain on urination, penile drip/discharge in 50 percent of men
Syphilis	majority asymptomatic

Parasitic
Trichomonas	majority asymptomatic
Pubic Lice	**itchiness**

18. IF STD SYMPTOMS DO APPEAR, WHAT ARE THEY?

Viral

HPV	New wart or mole-like growth; cervical, vaginal, penile, anal or oral mass
HSV1 – oral	Facial, nasal, lip or mouth (initial attack only) shallow sore(s)/irritation(s)
HSV1 – genital	Genital or buttock sore(s)/irritation(s)
HSV2	Genital or buttock sore(s)/irritation(s)
Hep C	Fever, fatigue, nausea, yellow eyes and skin
Hep B	Fever, fatigue, nausea, yellow eyes and skin
HIV	Fever, sore throat, rash

Bacterial

Chlamydia	Genital or anal discharge
Mycoplasma	Genital or anal discharge
Gonorrhea	Genital or anal discharge
Syphilis	Genital, anal or oral sore or body rash

Parasitic

Trichomonas	Genital discharge
Pubic Lice	Itching, tiny red skin spots (bites)

19. STD INCUBATION PERIOD: IF STD SYMPTOMS DO APPEAR, HOW LONG AFTER CONTACT?

Viral

HPV	90 – 8000 (20 years)
HSV1 – oral	3 - 12
HSV1 – genital	3 - 12
HSV2	3 - 12
Hep C	60 - 90
Hep B	60 - 90
HIV	14 - 60

Bacterial

Chlamydia	7 - 28
Mycoplasma	7 - 28
Gonorrhea	2 - 6
Syphilis	10 - 90

Parasitic

Trichomonas	5 - 28
Pubic Lice	7 - 14

20. WHAT ARE POSSIBLE STD COMPLICATIONS?

Consequences of no treatment:

Viral

HPV	Low Risk Strains: warts
	High Risk Strains: cancer (cervical, vaginal, vulvar, penile, anal or oral)
	1 percent lifetime risk HPV associated cancer
HSV1 – oral	Recurrent oral sores
HSV1 – genital	Recurrent genital sores (less frequent than HSV2)
HSV2	One in ten get recurrent genital sores, one in three hundred get severe recurrent attacks
Hep C	25 percent (if adult onset) liver cancer, cirrhosis
Hep B	2 percent (if adult onset) or 35 percent (if childhood onset) chance liver cancer, cirrhosis
HIV	99 percent chance AIDS (after 5-10 years) and death (2-3 years after onset AIDS)

Bacterial

Chlamydia	10 percent chance of infertility; increased ovarian cancer risk, miscarriage, pre-term birth or tubal pregnancy. Blindness in newborn
Mycoplasma	Infertility, tubal pregnancy
	Miscarriage or pre-term birth if pregnant
Gonorrhea	Infertility, tubular pregnancy, arthritis
	Miscarriage or pre-term birth if pregnant, blindness in newborn
Syphilis	33 percent chance severe internal disease, especially heart or brain;
	Miscarriage, preterm or stillbirth if pregnant, severe birth defects in infant

Parasitic

Trichomonas	Increased risk for HIV, complications in pregnancy
Pubic Lice	Chronic itching

STDs	Urge	Discharge**	Pain with urination
Chlamydia	(+++++)	scant, thin, clear-whitish	(++)
Mycoplasma	(+++)	scant, clear-whitish	(++)
Gonorrhea	(++)	scant→profuse, yellow-green	(+++)
Trichomonas	(++)	scant→profuse, clear-white	(+)
HSV1	(+)	rare	(+++++)
HSV2	(+)	rare	(+++++)
Adenovirus	(+)	scant, clear	(+++++)
Bowel bacteria	(+)	rare	(++)

Non-STD "Pretenders":

long duration sex	(++++)	none	(+)
bacterial UTI	(++)	none	(+++)
psychological	(++)	none	(+)
prostatitis	(++)	scant, white	(++)
instrumentation	(+)	cant, clear	(++++)
drug/chemical/irritant	(rare)	scant, clear	(+++)
urethral stricture	(rare)	none	(++)
doxycycline^^	(+/-)	none	(+/-)

** discharge: look for tip of penis crusting or underwear staining (see WHITE UNDERWEAR test, page 163)

^^ discomfort on urination is an unusual complication of doxycycline treatment; When it happens, it makes patients nervous that the STD is not getting better!

STD Causes: Other Comments

Chlamydia	"School girl" STD; beware of co-infections with other STDs
Mycoplasma	As common as chlamydia, many doctors unaware accurate test is now available
Gonorrhea	Beware! Some strains are resistant to the usual antibiotics
Trichomonas	More common than you think, uncertain if always sexually transmitted
HSV1	A "new" adult onset epidemic now that childhood infection less common
	Oral sex is a risk factor
HSV2	Lesions inside urethra can't be seen - but sure can be felt
Adenovirus	Tends to occur in the fall/winter, spread via oral sex, genital touching
Bowel bacteria	Rare. Occasionally an issue in persons engaging in anal sex

Non-STD "Pretenders:"

Long duration sex	Discomfort mild and transient
Bacterial UTI	Causes of up to 6 percent of urethritis cases
Psychological	Often associated with sex outside of monogamous long-standing relationship, or encounters with partners with unusual practices; almost always includes feelings of strong guilt
Prostatitis	May be associated with perineal (behind scrotum) pain
Instrumentation	Tip of urethra often irritated after catherization, insertion of devices during sex play
Chemical irritants	Exposure to douches, spermicides, insertion of drugs like cocaine or meth into penis urethral stricture (partial closure and scarring of urethral opening); possible complication of an untreated bacterial STD

22. IS VAGINAL DISCHARGE AN STD OR AN STD PRETENDER?

(Remember! Most sexually transmitted infections cause no vaginal discharge)

STD Causes: **If Discharge Present, Discharge Consistency:**

STD Causes:	If Discharge Present, Discharge Consistency:
Chlamydia	Thin
Gonorrhea	Thick, pus-like
Mycoplasma	Thin
Trich	Whitish, may be profuse, bubbly

Non-STD "Pretenders:"

Healthy*	A small amount of vaginal discharge is normal normal discharge increases with birth control and pregnancy
Psychologic	"Healthy" discharge; often underlying anxiety disorder
Allergic	Thin, may be itchy
Bacterial Vaginosis	Fishy odor, thin
Yeast	Itchy, thick, cottage cheese consistency
Chemical (suppositories)	Thin
Lichen Planus	Thin discharge, associated with open lesions

* normal healthy discharge consists of cervical secretions plus sloughed vaginal lining cells and adherent bacteria

23. ARE VISIBLE GENITAL SORES AN STD OR AN STD PRETENDER?

STD Causes

HSV1	HSV1 and HSV2 visually identical – genital, buttock or low lumbar region rash
HSV2	Red dots progress to clusters of blisters, then healing scabs
Syphilis	Painless ulcers, usually no lymph nodes
Chancroid	Painful ulcers and lymph nodes
LGV	Ulcers transient, tender lymph nodes

Non-STD "Pretenders:"

Shingles (Herpes Zoster)	Can look like HSV rash, but it only rarely reoccurs in same location. Often mis-diagnosed instead of herpes, partly to avoid patient "melt-down"
Folliculitis	Red small bumps, infected hair follicles
Acne	Clogged skin oil glands causing bumps, sores and cysts
Lichen Planus	Red, painful, burning open sores, occasional vaginal discharge
Pemphigus	Autoimmune blistering disease, often presents on labial lips
Bug bites	Discrete itchy, red puncture sites
Trauma	Often linear cuts or scratches
Drug reactions	Typically, itchy, may have blistering phase
Cancer	May present as open ulcers

STD	Pain	Type of rectal fluid
Chlamydia	(++)	Thin
Gonorrhea	(+)	Pus
Mycoplasma	(+)	Thin
HSV1/HSV2	(++)	Thin, occasionally thick or bloody
LGV (rare)	(+)	Thin, may be bloody

Non-STD "Pretenders:"

Diarrhea (viral)	(+/-)	Watery diarrhea
Bacterial proctitis	(+/-)	Watery diarrhea
Ulcerative Colitis	(+/-)	Urge to defecate with only mucous discharge Stools may be bloody
Crohns Disease	(+/-)	As above
Mechanical irritation	(+)	None
Chemical irritations	(+)	Thin, itchy
Rectal abscess	(+++)	None or pus if abscess ruptures
Hemorrhoids	(+/-)	None but anal mass may bleed bright red blood
Fissures	(++)	None
Fistulas	(+/-)	Thin or pus or stool from tract opening off to the side of anus

STD: Diagnosis and Treatment

Viral

HPV	High risk HPV testing (95 - 99%) (more accurate for cervical cancer detection than PAP screening) (95%)
HSV1 – oral	HSV1 DNA oral swab (99%) or visual findings plus antibody blood test (95 - 99%)
HSV1 – genital	HSV1 DNA genital swab (99%) or visual findings plus antibody blood test (95 - 99%)
HSV2	HSV2 DNA genital swab (99%) or antibody blood test (confirm with 2nd test) (95 - 99%)
Hep C	Antibody blood test (confirm with 2nd blood DNA test) (99%)
Hep B	Antibody blood test (confirm with 2nd blood DNA test) (99%)
HIV	Antibody blood test (confirm with 2nd blood DNA test) (99.9%)

Bacterial

Chlamydia	DNA urine or vaginal/oral/rectal swab test (98 - 99%)
Mycoplasma	DNA urine or vaginal/oral/rectal swab test (98 - 99%)
Gonorrhea	DNA urine or vaginal/oral/rectal swab test (98 - 99%)
Syphilis	Antibody blood test (confirm with 2nd specific treponemal test) (99%)

Parasitic

Trichomonas	DNA urine or swab test (98 - 99%)
Pubic Lice	Visualization

26. STD INCUBATION PERIOD: HOW LONG AFTER EXPOSURE DO STD TESTS TURN POSITIVE? (GENETIC VS. ANTIBODY TESTS)

Viral

HPV	90 (genetic#)
HSV1 – oral	14 (genetic*), 30 - 45 (antibody)
HSV1 – genital	14 (genetic*), 30 - 45 (antibody)
HSV2	14 (genetic*), 30 - 45 (antibody)
Hep C	30 - 60 (antibody)
Hep B	30 - 60 (antibody)
HIV	14 (genetic), 30 - 90 (antibody)

Bacterial

Chlamydia	5 (genetic)
Mycoplasma	5 (genetic)
Gonorrhea	5 (genetic)
Syphilis	21-42 (antibody)

Parasitic

Trichomonas	5 (genetic)
Pubic Lice	7-14 (visual)

\# Genetic tests, which directly detect the pathogen's DNA in the blood stream, turn "positive" faster than antibody tests, which require time for the body's immune system to react to the various pathogens.

* Genetic (swab) testing not generally available for HSV1 or HSV2 unless visible lesions are present.

27. BEST STD TREATMENTS?

Viral

HPV	Detection and removal of warts or pre-cancerous and cancerous lesions
HSV1 – oral	Antivirals, periodically for suppression
HSV1 – genital	Antivirals, daily or periodic suppression
HSV2	Antivirals, daily or periodic suppression
Hep C	Antivirals (8 - 12-week oral course), curative
Hep B	Antivirals, lifelong suppression
HIV	Antivirals, lifelong suppression

Bacterial

Chlamydia	Antibiotics, curative
Mycoplasma	Antibiotics, curative
Gonorrhea	Antibiotics (by injection), curative
Syphilis	Antibiotics (by injection), curative

Parasitic

Trichomonas	Antibiotics, curative
Pubic Lice	Cream, curative

STD Prevention

Viral

HPV	Vaccination ages 12-14. Vaccine works at all ages – the vaccine proportionally less effective as individuals more sexually active
HSV1 – oral	Condoms, antivirals, education, openness
HSV1 – genital	Condoms, antivirals, education, openness
HSV2	Condoms, antivirals, education, openness
Hep C	No needle sharing
Hep B	Vaccination at birth
HIV	Antiviral PrEP, PEP, condoms

Bacterial

Chlamydia	Condoms, PrEP antibiotics
Mycoplasma	Condoms
Gonorrhea	Condoms
Syphilis	Condoms, PrEP antibiotics

Parasitic

Trichomonas	Condoms
Pubic Lice	Pubic hair removal

29. WHAT STD SCREEN IS "COMPLETE"?

SCREENING STD TESTS

Blood	Cash Price
HSV — Herpes Select (HSV1/2 antibodies)	46
HIV — HIV antigen/Antibody, 4th Generation	22
Hepatitis C — Hep C Surface Antibody	16
Hepatitis B — Hep B Surface Antibody and antigen	13
Syphilis — RPR	4

Urine or Vaginal Swab (If Exposure)	
Gonorrhea — RNA Amplified	78
Chlamydia — RNA Amplified	78
Mycoplasma — by PCR	80
Trichomonas — DNA Amplified	24

Throat Swab (If Exposure)	
Gonorrhea — RNA Amplified	78
Chlamydia — RNA Amplified	78

Rectal Swab (If Exposure)	
Gonorrhea — RNA Amplified	78
Chlamydia — RNA Amplified	78

Cervical Testing	
High Risk HPV screen	75
PAP smear	150

Other	
HPV — Anal or oral high risk HPV screen (Non FDA approved)	75
Pubic Lice — Visual Identification	0
UTI — Urine Analysis	20
Candidiasis — Vaginal Discharge KOH Test	15
Bacterial Vaginosis — Vaginal Discharge eval	25

*Not yet validated; not yet recommended for routine diagnosis

CONFIRMATORY TESTS

	Cash Price
Western Blot	226
HSV1/2 antibodies (U of Washington)	
HIV RNA quantitative	126
Hep C quant PCR	61
Hep B DNA quant PCR	61
Treponemal EIA	30
Culture	40

30. Best STD Prevention Plan for Heterosexuals (Married or Single) with Multiple Partners?

Baseline prevention:
1. Education: stigma vs. facts.
2. If you are positive for a lifelong viral STD, fully educate yourself. Stigma and STD phobia is perpetuated by ignorance and fear. Don't be part of that vicious cycle.
3. If you have a new STD:
   - notify recent partners. If you are not freaked out or ashamed, your partner will likewise process the information calmly.
   - get your doctor to treat your recent partners with the appropriate treatment(s) without a doctor visit (expedited treatment!)
   - partner(s) cannot be treated without consent – i.e. you can't sneak an antibiotic into your spouse's coffee!

4. The only times it makes sense to immediately run into your doctor's office "the morning after":
   - if you had unprotected sex with someone with a known STD
   - if you had unprotected sex with someone with a high risk of being HIV positive
   - if you have symptoms consistent with an STD
   - if you are uncertain about how to best protect your spouse or "other" partners after an out of relationship high risk sex encounter
   - an out of relationship sex encounter if your regular partner is pregnant
   - the risk of an unwanted pregnancy can be handled with OTC Plan B
5. Better to test yourself and future partner(s) "beforehand" rather than "afterward."
6. It takes a week to several months after contact before STD tests turn positive (the "window period").
7. If your STD tests are "all" good — be aware of the "window period" — and the fact that most doctors don't test for HPV, HSV, trichomonas or mycoplasma.
8. Noncoital behaviors (mutual masturbation, oral sex) is low risk for most but not all STDs.
9. Partner selection: a lot of time is spent choosing a life partner, precious little on casual partner(s) who are at far higher risk of STD.
10. Vaccinations (if not adequately vaccinated):
    - HPV-9 vaccination series (even if older than 26 years of age)
    - Hep A vaccination series
    - Hep B vaccination series
    - Meningococcal
    - Shingles (optional if you have symptomatic HSV1/2, anecdotal reports of occasional benefit)
11. Circumcision.
12. Premenopausal: birth control pills do not prevent STDs (use BCP's plus condom).
13. Postmenopausal females: topical estrogen cream protective against sex associated UTIs, perhaps also STDs.
14. No cigarettes - even several/day are toxic.
15. No excessive alcohol.
16. Good oral hygiene.
17. Optimal fitness - body fat diet and sleep – that in turn optimizes the disease fighting immune system.

Pre-sex prevention:

18. Avoid pubic skin shaving 48 hrs prior to sex.
19. Pre-Exposure Prophylaxis (PrEP) for at risk sex:
    - Truvada (HIV exposure)
    - Doxycycline (Chlamydia/syphilis exposure)
20. Limit recreational drugs and alcohol pre-sex (increased STD risk).

Game-time prevention:

21. Partner discussion: Last STD testing? Contraception? Sexual preferences?
22. Disclose your STD status to partner(s).
23. Discuss condoms - be positive! "Condom makes me feel better. I orgasm better knowing I'm protected!"
24. Optimize your use of condoms (Lelo Hex condom may be less prone to slip off or rupture).
25. Avoid oil-based lubricants/medications - i.e. hand creams, baby oil, Vaseline products or medicine like miconazole vaginal cream that can disrupt latex and weaken condoms.

Post-sex protection:

26. Post Exposure Prophylaxis (PEP) (for HIV, chlamydia and syphilis).
27. Plan B if condom-less vaginal sex (premenopausal woman).
28. STD testing - after condom-less sex with untested outside partner(s):
    - If symptoms, get immediate testing
    - If no symptoms, wait 4 weeks and get full STD screen before resuming condom-less sex with your other partner(s). As described previously, regular STD checks are needed even with religious use of condoms. STDs can still be transmitted around a properly placed condom – especially HPV, HSV, pubic lice and syphilis.

Testing for individuals with multiple anonymous partners:

HPV	Females begin PAPs at age 21 (every 3 years);
	HPV screening begins at 30 (every 5 years)
	Males and females: vaccinate with Gardasil 9
Hep C	One-time blood test only for those born in the 50s or 60s
Hep A or B	One-time blood test, vaccinate if unprotected

Yearly blood and urine (swab) testing (every three to six months if multiple anonymous partners):

1. HSV1/HSV2	Blood tests	only if no past history of infection
2. HIV	Blood tests	only if no past history of infection
3. Syphilis	Blood tests	
4. Chlamydia	Urine (swab) test	
5. Trichomonas	Urine (swab) test	
6. Mycoplasma	Urine (swab) test	
7. Gonorrhea	Urine (swab) test	
8. Pubic Lice	Visual exam	

31. Best STD Prevention Plan for Pregnant Women and Their Babies?

Baseline prevention:

1. Education: It's all about the baby's health!
2. Pre-pregnancy vaccinations.
3. Noncoital behaviors (mutual masturbation, oral sex) is low risk for most but not all STDs.
4. Ideal health (especially pertaining to immune function) which is dependent on: proper diet, exercise and sleep.
5. No cigarettes (even several/day are toxic), no alcohol, good oral hygiene, and be fit.
6. Full preventative treatment if partner(s) positive for any STDs.
7. Screen for STD's early in pregnancy baby's' health:

• HPV	Continue routine cervical cancer screening	
• Hep B	Blood tests	if no past history of infection
• HSV1/HSV2	Blood tests	if no past history of infection
• HIV	Blood tests	if no past history of infection
• Syphilis	Blood tests	
• Chlamydia	Urine test	
• Gonorrhea	Urine test	
• Mycoplasma	Urine test	

8. Repeat STD testing each 3 months if any high-risk sexual exposures or either partner has out of relationship sex.
9. Highly effective treatments exist for averting fetal damage from syphilis, chlamydia, and gonorrhea.
10. Highly effective preventative treatments exist for averting fetal damage from HIV, Hep B and HSV.

Pre-sex prevention:

11. Avoid pubic skin shaving 48 hrs prior to sex.
12. If male partner HIV positive on anti-HIV medication, PrEP (Truvada) may be added for pregnant women for "safer" impregnation. PrEP is safe in pregnancy.

Game-time prevention:

13. Once pregnant, if in real doubt about your partner(s) STD status, use condoms pending testing.

Post-sex protection:

14. PEP (HIV, HSV) in certain circumstances may be indicated – doxycycline for prophylaxis syphilis and chlamydia is contraindicated during pregnancy (tetracyclines stain developing teeth).
15. C-Section may be necessary for a new HSV infection near delivery. Repeat STD testing as needed based on symptoms.

32. Best STD Prevention Plan for Virgins Considering 1st Sexual Encounter?

Baseline prevention:
1. Education: fact vs. stigma.
2. Noncoital behaviors (mutual masturbation, oral sex) is low risk for most but not all STDs.
3. Test potential initial partner(s): full specific prevention if partner STD positive.
4. If partner STD testing "all OK," remember usually HPV, HSV, trichomonas and mycoplasma not tested.
5. Vaccinations: HPV-9 (update even if you had the childhood HPV-4), Hep B, Hep A, meningococcal.
6. Circumcision.
7. Ideal health (especially pertaining to immune function).
8. No cigarettes, avoid excessive alcohol, maintain good oral hygiene and be fit (sex occasionally causes heart attacks or sudden death).
9. Have solid pregnancy prevention method: long-acting birth control or birth control pills plus condom.

Pre-sexual contact prevention:
10. No pubic skin shaving 48 hrs prior to sex.
11. No need for PrEP if initial partner tested.
12. Limit recreational drugs and alcohol; their use prior to sex increases STD risk.

Game-time prevention:
13. Talk to partner(s): Any communicable disease symptoms? Last STD/HIV testing? Contraception?
    Sexual orientation? Realize that answers cannot be fully believed
14. Avoid oil-based lubricants/medications – i.e. hand creams, Vaseline products
    or meds like miconazole vaginal cream that can disrupt latex and weaken condoms.
15. Use condoms.

Post-sex protection:
16. Post intercourse urination, showering with soap may possibly help
17. No need for PEP if initial partner tested
18. Plan B if any unprotected sex
19. STD testing as needed for suspicious symptoms
20. Routine testing post exposure not needed if initial partner tested.

STD screen for virgin: One-time testing for

HSV1	Blood tests
Hep A and B	Blood tests, vaccinate if unprotected

33. Best STD Prevention Plan for Men Who Have Sex with Men (MSM) and Have Multiple Partners?

Baseline prevention:
1. Education: stigma vs. facts.
2. MSM are at high risk of contracting STDs, including HIV, HSV, syphilis, gonorrhea and chlamydia.
3. Test yourself regularly at all anatomic sites (throat, urine, rectum and blood).
4. Encourage partners to test exposed regularly: get full treatment if STD positive.
5. Remember, it takes at least three weeks to several months before STD tests turn positive.
6. If your STD tests are "all" good, be aware HPV, HSV, trichomonas and mycoplasma are often not tested
7. Vaccinations: HPV-9 (even if older than 26), Hep A, Hep B and meningococcal.
8. Circumcision.
9. Ideal health, especially pertaining to immune function which is dependent on: proper diet, exercise and sleep.
10. No cigarettes (even several/day are toxic), no excessive alcohol, maintain good oral hygiene.

Pre-sex prevention:
11. Avoid pubic skin shaving 48 hrs prior to sex.
12. If multiple untested partners: use HIV Prep (Truvada) daily.
13. If multiple untested partners and no condom: Use chlamydia and syphilis PrEP (doxycycline 100 mg daily or 200 mg after sex).
14. If multiple partners, no condom and HSV negative: consider unproven HSV PrEP (Valtrex).
15. Limit recreational drugs and alcohol pre-sex (increased STD risk).

Game-time prevention:
16. Partner discussion: Any communicable disease symptoms? Last HIV/STD testing? Remember answers cannot be fully believed.
17. Disclose your HIV/STD status to partner(s).
18. Use condoms (Lelo Hex condom may be less prone to slip off or rupture).
19. Avoid oil-based lubricants/medications – i.e. hand creams, baby oil, Vaseline products that can weaken latex condoms.
20. Use plenty of water-based (or silicone) lubrication.

Post-sex protection:
21. Post intercourse urination may possibly help.
22. PEP (post exposure prophylaxis) (HIV, chlamydia and syphilis) if neither PrEP or condom used.
23. STD testing if any suspicious symptoms.
24. Expedited treatment both partners if STD identified.

Routine STD screening for MSM with multiple partners:
Test each 3 to 6 months (3 months if using PrEP):

HSV1 and HSV2	Blood tests	if no past history of infection
HIV	Blood tests	if no past history of infection
Hep C	Blood tests	
Syphilis	Blood tests	
Chlamydia	Urine and rectal	
Mycoplasma	Urine tests	
Gonorrhea	Urine, rectal and throat test	
Pubic Lice	Visual Exam	
HPV	No oral testing at this time, HPV 9 vaccination if indicated (up to 65 years old) Some in community do rectal "PAP" smears but like the oral testing, benefits have not yet been established	
Hep A and B	One-time blood test, vaccinate if unprotected; high risk HPV screen is a more plausible cancer screen, but also untested - potential benefits not established	

34. Are STDs Being Properly Addressed by the Law?

In the 80's – the heyday of herpes fear and loathing (before HIV gave persons with herpes a new perspective) – some jilted lovers were extracting revenge by suing the ex for emotional and physical distress for passing on a STD. The first highly publicized multimillion-dollar case was filed by a Comedy Store employee against Robin William for giving her herpes. In many cases, the person being sued was as clueless as the suing party about STD detection and prevention. However, California law states "it is illegal to knowingly or recklessly transmit a sexually transmitted disease." So, once an STD is known, a failure to disclose invites legal liability – and bad press!

The woman acknowledged she never asked Williams whether he had a sexually transmitted disease and that the actor never denied he had herpes. She also said she had unprotected sex with at least eight other lovers before and after Williams and had never asked any of them whether they were infected.

"Incurable" STDs, namely genital HSV, HPV and HIV, must be in play if the plaintiff hopes to get a lawyer on contingency, because it's not about winning, it's about provable damages. An ex could win a lawsuit based on an easily treatable STD such as gonorrhea, syphilis, or chlamydia, but the damages might not amount to more than the cost of a one-dose antibiotic treatment.

Step one is convincing a jury that a reasonable person would have abstained from sex unless first informing his or her partner of the risk of STD infection. Curiously, negligence does not require intent, so ,an ex can still be found responsible for giving a partner an STD and responsible to pay reasonable damages even *if a condom was used*!

A more aggressive strategy involves suing the ex for sexual battery, basically claiming that not disclosing his or her STD status was tantamount to rape or nonconsensual sex. So, if a man knew he was infected with herpes and failed to tell his partner, her consent for that sexual encounter is effectively wiped out. As with negligence, the ex need not have wanted to infect you with his or her STD. This aggressive interpretation of the law only requires that he or she intended to have sex with you without disclosing his or her dangerous STD status.

Proving liability in states which criminalize sex when a known STD was not fully disclosed is straightforward. For example, in many states, it is a felony to have sex without disclosing a known HIV positive condition. Here's where landmark advances in HIV treatment are intersecting with archaic 1980's law: Is it reasonable to charge, convict and incarcerate an HIV infected person with a felony for failing to disclose HIV status pre-intercourse if that individual is fully treated with anti-retroviral meds (HIV viral load count <20), who CDC experts believe has a zero-transmission risk?

The state of California recently took an exemplary step – in late 2017, state law was changed so that it is no longer a felony to sexually transmit HIV. The hope is that this change will encourage all individuals at risk to test for HIV without the worry of possible future criminal repercussions. The #MeToo campaign, which has targeted sexual harassment in all walks of life, gives us multiple opportunities to make consensual sex emotionally, medically and legally safer.

Prior to initiating sexual relations, partners need to have an open discussion and, optimally, a physical transfer of information concerning STDs. This communication becomes an informed consent on multiple levels. Ultimately, the law puts the full burden of disclosure on the individual with "known" STDs — however, in the spirit of honesty, equality and transparency — both partners should physically exchange their most recent complete STD labs and vaccine record results prior to intimacy.

Usher Raymond's recent legal woes illustrate many of these issues. As of June, 2018, he is being sued in California Superior court for purportedly not disclosing his genital herpes infection to three past sexual partners (one claims he spread his herpes to her, the other two accusers are not infected with herpes). In California "it is illegal to knowingly or recklessly transmit a sexually transmitted disease."

It would seem straightforward to reject the claims from the two individuals who are herpes negative – they did not get herpes transmitted to them. However, as previously mentioned, new aggressive legal interpretations of the law can be used to accuse Usher of sexual battery, asserting the non-disclosure of his STD status invalidated his partners consent prior to their hook-up.

Where are the battle lines in this all-out legal war? Usher's lawyers could look carefully at the accusers' medical histories. Were they positive for HPV? Chlamydia? Yeast infections? For instance, they can claim the female partner did not reveal her positive PAP smear. HPV infection is orders of magnitude more medically dangerous than herpes… do you see how ugly it can get when you bring lawyers into the bedroom?

The individual claiming, she is herpes positive faces a difficult hurdle proving her herpes was in fact transmitted from Usher. Usher has apparently settled a past herpes transmission law suit with an individual for 1.1 million and medical expenses where it was stated he got a herpes diagnosis in 2010 - but does he really have herpes? Many individuals are given an incorrect diagnosis (based on a false positive herpes test). If he does in fact have accurate testing confirming herpes, his accusers still need to prove he gave them his exact herpes "strain": herpes needs to be cultured from each person in question and compared – a difficult and often impossible scientific undertaking. Women are twice as likely as men to have herpes so it would not be unusual for Usher's accusers to have independently picked up herpes from prior partners.

Understandably, I have heard financial advisors for celebrities with wealth, (i.e. sports stars and successful musicians) beg their clients to never get a potentially incriminating STD test. These highly publicized cases can have undesirable effects (the law of unintended consequences), potentially resulting in more STD transmission by encouraging young sexually active individuals to never test as a means of lowering their legal liability.

35. Can We Eliminate STDs ...Totally?!?

1. Education - let's work to destigmatize STDs, especially herpes and HIV.
   a. Understand origin of illogical hysteria – for example herpes simplex
      i. Full education on exactly what a typical herpes infection typically does (serious outbreaks very rare)
      ii. Full education on the less than 1 percent who get significant herpes symptoms
2. Detection - Declare September as "National STD Check-Up Month" to identify the large pool of symptomless "STD carriers" and stop the vicious cycle.
   a. Place STD same-day testing and treatment in every high school and require students to test each fall
   b. Support affordable online home-based STD testing
   c. Ensure annual physician-initiated syphilis and chlamydia screening in recommended groups – MSM, pregnant women, all sexually active women less than 25 years of age (over one million American women under 25 currently have a symptom-less chlamydia infection)
3. Treatment
   a. Treat all infected persons and partners
   b. Detecting and treating STDs is the best STD prevention! We have to as a country wrap our collective mind around this fact.
4. Prevention.
   a. Provide free condoms in schools
   b. Teach kids how to properly use condoms
   c. Require HPV vaccination for 7th grade entry
   d. As appropriate, utilize pre and post sex drugs that eliminate or limit STD transmission
5. Research.
   a. Invest in syphilis, gonorrhea and chlamydia vaccine research
   b. Accelerate herpes vaccine development
   c. Study Valtrex taken prophylactically for HSV prevention
6. Political.
   a. Legalize sex work
   b. Require physician and patient notification of past partners when STDs are identified
   c. Properly fund public health agencies

These actions could essentially eliminate chlamydia, mycoplasma, gonorrhea, syphilis, trichomonas and pubic lice while halting the future spread of Hep C, HIV and to a lesser extent HSV.